BELLY
FAT
FREE

BELLY FAT FREE

Liberate Yourself From Obesity
Additives and Get a Flat Belly Fast

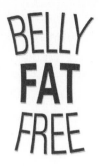

BELLY FAT FREE

Liberate Yourself From Obesity
Additives and Get a Flat Belly Fast

By Josh Bezoni

Belly Fat Free LLC

The Belly Fat Free Program is intended for healthy men and women ages 18 and older. This program is solely for information and educational purposes and is not medical advice. Please be sure to consult your doctor before starting a new diet or exercise program, particularly if you suffer from any medical condition or have any symptoms that may require medical treatment.

The individuals featured in this book are some of our most successful customers. They achieved extraordinary success by following a reduced-calorie diet described in the *Belly Fat Free* book ("BFF"); some also did regular exercise, as recommended in the book. Because individuals differ, the results you will achieve on the BFF program may differ from those achieved by others who followed the same program. Most people who buy *Belly Fat Free* do not follow it, so they lose little if any weight. Prior to the publication of this book, 108 people who followed the Belly Fat Free program for 12 weeks as part of our "BFF Challenge" reported their results to us. According to those reports, those people lost an average of 20 pounds in 12 weeks.

To the men and women throughout this great country who do their very best to consistently evolve and improve—to transform—while overcoming life's obstacles and challenges along the way. You are my inspiration.

Acknowledgments

I would like to begin by thanking my parents for teaching me that hard work, humor, and helping others can take you far in life; my sisters Molly and Mandy for keeping me in line and setting a good example (we need more mothers and teachers like you); all of my nieces and nephews for showing me the true meaning of joy; and Kim Eschner for her unyielding support and encouragement throughout the years. I love you all more than ice cream!

I also wish to express my deep appreciation to Vicky Grossie for her relentless dedication; Dean Graziosi for providing a vehicle to get this message out to America; Joe Polish for generously sharing his vast wisdom throughout the years and for introducing me to everyone and their dog (literally); and to so many mentors, most of whom I've only met through their written words.

I also thank Meredith Mooney for her research and writing abilities; the entire team at BellyFatFree.com for helping to bring this vision to life on all levels (especially Lisa Liddy and Gary Crump for their design skills); and my editors, Nikki Van Noy and Judy Wilson, for their attention to detail. And finally, last but certainly not least, I would like to extend my deepest respect and admiration to the men and women who are featured in the pages of this book. These inspiring folks have made incredible transformations despite the adversity and obstacles they encountered along the way. They are a great inspiration to me, and I thank them from the bottom of my heart.

Contents

Belly Fat Free

Join our free BFF online community at www.BellyFatFree.com

BFF Success Story
Tina: A Mother Fights for Her Children

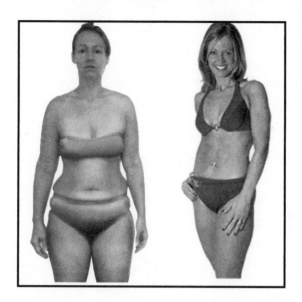

Tina White, a 35-year-old mother of two, had tried so many different diets over the years, and she was wary of being let down yet again. The last thing she needed was another disappointment.

She also had a habit of procrastinating. So although she had heard about the Belly Fat Free Program™, she kept putting it off. It was easy to make excuses about why she couldn't do it right now: she told herself her weight wasn't really all that bad, that she didn't have the time, that she'd start later. She lied to herself over and over again.

Then one day, she looked at her 10-year-old son and 9-year-old daughter, and it hit her like a Mack truck. Her children were following in her footsteps and, from the looks of things, that meant they were on the road to becoming very unhappy with their bodies. They spent too much time sitting. Between schoolwork, reading, watching TV, and playing video games, there just wasn't much real activity. To compound the problem, they ate too many empty calories…and it was starting to show. Scared, Tina knew she had to take action to prevent her children from falling victim to a fat lifestyle. It was time to stop procrastinating and to start getting her family on a healthier path.

Once Tina got fired up about her goal, there was no stopping her. Although her lightbulb moment happened right before Thanksgiving, she didn't use that as an excuse to stall. Tina was done procrastinating.

It didn't take long to discover that Belly Fat Free was different from all the diets Tina had tried in the past. She explains, "What I love about Belly Fat Free is that it's not overwhelming, it's not too strict, and it's very easy…even with a busy schedule like mine. Literally, you start where you're at and then you evolve along the way. When you adopt the right mindset, you shed your old bad habits. It's so liberating. The ugly fat melts off, and people can't help but notice the wonderful changes."

Tina's friends can't get over how great she looks, and there's a good reason why. **According to the scale Tina lost 35 pounds and her love handles vanished (not to mention those 30 inches that melted off).** But the thing is, she actually lost more than 35 pounds of fat, because she also put on attractive, lean muscle at the same time—completely transforming her body in the process. Best of all, Tina knows that she's now setting a good example for her children.

It will come as no surprise that today Tina looks great in a swimsuit and can literally wear whatever she wants. Not only are Tina's friends noticing her new body, but even strangers come up and give her compliments. Not to mention that Tina's relationship with her husband Neil has never been stronger. Her message to each and every person struggling with weight issues is that they can change their bodies and their lives…just as she did.

BFF Success Story
Mark: "I Finally Have A Life Again."

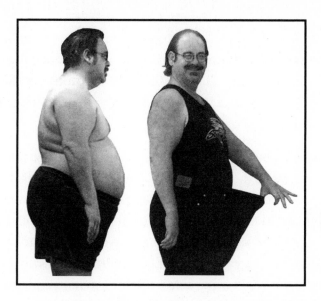

One of the most dramatic personal transformations I've ever witnessed is that of radio talk show host Mark Siffer. Mark began following Belly Fat Free when he was at a dangerously obese 361 pounds.

Within 12 months, Mark had lost 110 pounds, without dangerous prescription drugs or risky weight loss reduction surgery, all thanks to the principles in this book.

For Mark, the last straw was "When I had to buy size 56 pants, and the belt to go with them. I was really depressed. I just made a mental picture in my mind that I was going to be in one of those photos where I put on the 'fat pants' and showed the progress!" (You can see those very fat pants in the picture of Mark above.)

Mark had an incredible role model throughout the process, his sister Marcia Regan, a former winner in the BFF Challenge (see page 48). Mark saw how Marcia's life had changed—how

Belly Fat Free Success Story

much more pride, energy, and enthusiasm she had for life—and he wanted the same for himself. Mark knew that if Marcia could do it, he could too.

Mark first focused on lifestyle changes by removing belly-bulging obesity additives from his foods. He added high-quality supplements to his daily routine and began the habit of daily physical activity. As a result, Mark was soon down from a size 56 to a size 42.

Looking back, Mark feels that he was absolutely "dying of fat" before he made the decision to change. He says, "I really felt like if I did not change, I would be dead very soon. I hated myself. I would wait until dark to take the garbage out because I was embarrassed to be seen." Well, that's all changed. Now Mark finds staying at home boring, so you're more likely to find him hitting the open road (he put 7,000 miles on his Harley Davidson motorcycle this past year!), and he laughs about saving money on gasoline now that he's 110 pounds lighter. "Sometimes I think of so many things to do that I run out of time," Mark says. "I am not used to having all this energy. Life really is wonderful!"

CHAPTER 1

America...the Beautiful?

I would like to introduce you to the new symbol of American health and fitness...the Statue of Obesity.

Not as good looking as her sister, eh? For most of us, the

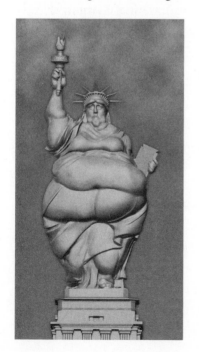

Statue of Liberty symbolizes freedom, opportunity, and hope for a brighter future. But unfortunately these days Lady Liberty no longer resembles her people. The sad truth is, today's typical American body—obese, unhealthy, and depressed—is the exact opposite of what this great statue was intended to represent.

Thanks to the help of a massive **obesity conspiracy** (and as you'll soon find out, no, this is not overly dramatic language) led by pharmaceutical drug giants, rip-off weight loss companies, and some shady food manufacturers who secretly hide obesity additives (covered in Chapter 4) in the foods we eat, many Americans have become trapped inside shells of fat that have stolen their physical freedom, health, and self-confidence. In short, their pursuit of happiness.

Believe it or not, 70 percent of American adults (more than 100 million men and women) are now overweight and are struggling with the most dangerous kind of fat—belly fat. Tragically, each year more than 350,000 of our friends and family members die from weight-related diseases, including certain cancers, diabetes, stroke, heart disease, and even depression (suicide). That's nearly *1,000 people every single day*—making obesity America's number one killer, surpassing even cigarette smoking.

And this is just the beginning. Millions more Americans are trapped in a life of quiet desperation. Many are hiding from the world, ashamed and embarrassed about their bodies and worried sick about their health. Make no mistake, these negative feelings affect every single aspect of our lives, from relationships to finances, to health and happiness.

As if all this isn't enough, it gets even worse—there's no end in sight. Childhood obesity is growing at an alarming rate, quadrupling over the past 30 years and destroying the health, confidence, and future happiness of more than 20 million American children in its wake.

Excess belly fat really has become the biggest threat to the health and security of Americans today. If we don't do something now, health care premiums will continue to skyrocket. In fact, many experts believe excess body fat will collapse the health care system *entirely* as our obese children grow up and get sick. After all, there is an 80 percent chance that an overweight child will become an overweight adult.

Maybe you can relate to this big fat problem?

If so, don't worry. Despite all this gloom and doom, there is *real* hope for a brighter future. In fact, I'd like to share it with you right now. It's a secret that more than 100,000 men and women are already using to lose that excess weight once and for all.

Believe it or not, you hold these secrets in your hands right now. I call them my Belly Fat Free (BFF) secrets.

Progressive doctors and nutritionists are recommending Belly Fat Free in record numbers because their patients don't have to turn their lives upside down to experience fast and extraordinary results. Get this: You don't even have to stop eating your favorite foods. And, no, you don't have to exercise 24/7 either.

I know, I know. It sounds too good to be true. But this is not another weight loss gimmick...and even better, it really is as simple as 1, 2, 3.

1. **Lose the additives.** Eat and drink less of the foods and beverages that contain deadly obesity additives (we'll discuss these in detail in Chapter 4), and replace them with safe and tasty versions of different brands of foods. Many of my students do *only* this and achieve a flat belly fast.

2. **It's all about timing and combining (optional).** When you eat and what you eat are extremely important when it comes to battling belly fat. Learn to eat the right foods at the right times throughout the day to naturally increase your fat- and calorie-burning metabolism. Not only do you get to keep eating the same amount of food, but sometimes you'll even be able to eat more.

3. **Move your body (optional).** If you want to burn away stubborn belly fat even faster, it's important to learn the

secrets to getting maximum results in minimum time from exercise. I'll show you how.

Doesn't sound too hard, huh? It gets even better. If you want even faster results, I'll demonstrate a simple five-minute BFF Transformation Program™ so easy you can do it while watching your favorite TV program. (A more advanced plan is also available in Chapter 9.)

In these pages, I'll also let you in on the truth about the Great American Obesity Conspiracy (see Chapter 4). Armed with this knowledge, you and your family can escape the sinister control of the weight loss rip-off artists, profit-hungry drug giants, and sneaky food manufacturers that all profit from keeping you and your loved ones overweight and unhealthy.

Make no mistake, Belly Fat Free (BFF) is a program you can follow for life. Through BFF I want us to become "best friends forever." And like any good friend I want what's best for you. That's why it's my goal to help you quickly achieve a new, head-turning body once and for all…without the yo-yo weight gain rebound so many people experience when following those restrictive diet programs of the past.

So now let me ask you: Wouldn't you like to join BFF to achieve a new, trim body and help us in our mission to slim down the Statue of Obesity, bringing the hope, happiness, and health back to our country once and for all?

If your answer is a resounding, "Yes!" you can join our fight against fat by donating your unwanted belly fat to our cause starting right now. It works like this: Follow the BFF Program outlined in this book. For every pound you report losing at our online support community BellyFatFree.com, we will remove a pound from the Statue of Obesity featured on our Web site.

Collectively, our goal is to help remove 100 tons of fat, blubber, and cellulite from the Statue of Obesity and to restore her to her rightful place as a symbol of freedom, pride, and hope for all Americans. Of course, you'll also be liberating yourself from unattractive and unhealthy fat while creating a future brimming with confidence, health, and happiness for you and your family.

And if all that's not enough motivation for you, we have tens of thousands of dollars in cash and prizes just waiting to be claimed by the men and women who undergo the most extraordinary transformations as part of our BFF Challenge™. (Be sure to visit BellyFatFree.com/Challenge for more information.)

There will never be a more perfect time than now to start your journey. Life is never going to be less busy. "Later" may never come. This is your big chance to finally live up to your true potential— not only to become happy, healthy, and confident but also to set an example for those you love the most.

Won't you join our mission to fight belly fat now? If so, hold on tight...because the adventure begins the moment you turn this page.

[Belly Fat Free Challenge: Void in CO, FL, IA, MD, VT, and outside the 50 United States and the District of Columbia, and where prohibited. Contest open only to persons who are both legal residents of one of the United States (including DC) and at least 18 years old at the beginning of the contest. For start and end dates of the contest and complete Official Rules, visit BellyFatFree.com/Challenge. Sponsor: Belly Fat Free, LLC, 7251 West Lake Mead Boulevard Ste 300, Las Vegas, NV 89128.]

BFF Success Story
Rita: Finally Free From Fat

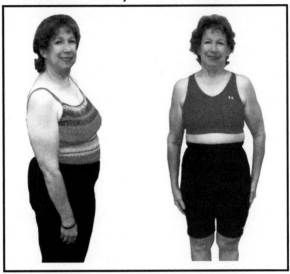

Rita Pilger, a 55-year-old mom from Arvada, Colorado, was born with a congenital dislocated hip. From ages one to five, she underwent multiple surgeries that included bone grafts, wire stitches, and bone wedges that were placed in her hip sockets—all accompanied by excruciating pain.

Every surgery ended in disappointment, as each one was never as successful as Rita had hoped. Rita recalls living in constant panic. As a child, she never knew when she would be whisked away to another "surprise" surgery that left her isolated and trapped in a body cast for months on end.

Understandably, her self-esteem was demolished and she felt she had little control over her life, because she had little control over her body and what was happening to her.

As Rita grew up, she went on to get married and have children. Looking back, she remembers times when her husband and children had to push her in a wheelchair and do the physical tasks she wished she could have done for them.

Decades later, when Rita needed a double hip replacement, her doctor issued a warning: "Try to get as thin as you can, because your new hips are delicate, and losing weight will be important for maintaining them." But the doctor didn't have any real advice on how to achieve this weight loss. Rita tried to lose weight, but the fad diets she tried only left her hungry, confused, and depressed before the surgery. As a result, she ended up feeding her emotions and gained 25 pounds.

Later, Rita's sister told her about **The Belly Fat Free Program** and showed her the Web site. Rita loved what she saw and knew it was for her. Rita's perseverance paid off when she ended up shedding **64 pounds and more than 40 inches of baggage** with BFF.

Rita likes to say she's lost "a yard of fat." She went from wearing size 18 jeans to size 6 petite. She used to dress only in dark "slimming" colors, but now she's enjoying bright, vibrant shades that match her mood—and all of her friends are noticing.

Getting into smaller clothes and feeling great isn't the only way Rita's life has changed. As she got into better shape, she felt she needed a more challenging exercise than the recumbent bike she owned, so she joined her local gym. Now she's employed there— something she wouldn't have predicted in a million years—and she's helping others lose belly fat just like she did.

Rita likes to challenge people with the question, "What's your reason for wanting to change?" What was her reason? "I wanted to be physically free," says Rita. "I spent so many years of my life trapped in body casts, and then I spent even more time trapped in a shell of body fat…I just wanted to be physically free and in control of my body for once in my life. That's what drove me and still drives me today."

Rita says, "After you figure out why you want to change, then you need to make an irrevocable decision to succeed, with a deadline. The best way to do that is to follow **Belly Fat Free**. It doesn't matter if you don't lose as fast as someone else. Just try it. It will change your life."

CHAPTER 2

Challenge Yourself to Change

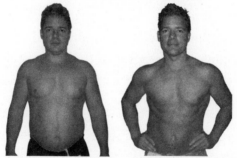

I lost 32 pounds following my Belly Fat Free Program; you can too!

As I stood looking at my reflection in the mirror I was defeated, broken, exhausted, and *beyond* depressed. My life had hit a point so low I could no longer see the light. I had lost my way, and everything seemed to be fading to black.

I had started a company—one I wasn't passionate about—and over the course of a few years, my lack of enthusiasm and poor judgment put me $150,000 in debt, $100,000 of which was on credit cards. Worry and uncertainty filled my every waking thought—and because I couldn't sleep at night, my misery was constant. Despite the fact that I had nothing but debt to show for it, I was a workaholic. It was almost all I did, all I thought about. It consumed my life. It consumed my soul.

As if all this wasn't enough, a long-term relationship ended badly at the same time. Looking back, it was a relationship that was anything but healthy. It was completely toxic and dysfunctional, inside and out, and it all came crashing down, leaving me feeling alone, isolated, and desperate. (Oh, if only I knew then what I know now.)

I was a prisoner by my own design—almost agoraphobic. There were periods when I would barely leave my house, consuming handfuls of anti-anxiety medications just to make it through the day. When I did go out, I was frequently riddled with stress-induced anger. During my early 20s I drank too much, got into bar fights, and made regular visits to the emergency room to get my face stitched up. Somehow I had stumbled onto a very dark path. I was a lost soul.

My mind and body were being poisoned with anxiety, negative thoughts, and destructive foods, causing toxic amounts of stress hormones to course through my veins. My joints were filled with so much inflammation I could barely move without experiencing pain. (It got so bad that I had two unnecessary surgeries on my left knee and right shoulder, neither of which were the same for years afterward.)

My hair was falling out from the worry. My mind was screaming for balance. I was like a zombie, hiding from my problems by sleeping and watching countless hours of TV. I put on more than 32 pounds of fat by feeding my emotions day in and day out— using food as a Band-Aid to mask my real problems. In short, I was self-destructing.

Although drugs and alcohol were not my addictions, I *was* an addict and my poisons of choice were certainly no better. I was addicted to obesity additives, stress, depression, inactivity, anger, and negativity. I was attracting into my life exactly what I thought about throughout each day. I had literally created my own hell.

Perhaps worst of all, I was ashamed of the person I saw looking back at me in the mirror. How could this have happened? How could I have let myself get to this point? Where had it all gone wrong? I used to be an athletic, successful, fun-loving person. I didn't recognize who I had become.

I was drowning in the coldest, iciest waters of life, gasping for air.

It was at that very moment that I finally confronted myself in the mirror and decided to change. To do whatever it took to transform myself from what I had become to what I *could* become. I decided to become more. I decided to live. After all, the alternative was unthinkable.

> I vowed to myself that I would look and feel like a new man in exactly 12 weeks.

But if I was going to live, I was going to live on my terms. I was going to fully engage life. I was going to be happy and fulfilled. I was going to live up to my potential. And I was going to treat life like the gift it truly is.

I would stop making excuses. I would stop being negative and toxic. I would start making my health and body a priority. I would help and encourage others. I would love and live as best I could.

Then and there in front of that mirror I vowed to myself that I would look and feel like a new man in exactly 12 weeks. With a newfound resolution, I then turned and walked away from the defeated reflection that had stared back at me for so long…for the very last time.

I began my transformation that very night by reclaiming control of my body. This consisted of nothing more than a 10-minute jog. It was all I could do. My knee and shoulder ached and there was a voice in my head screaming out to stop. I pushed forward anyway…and that, in and of itself, gave me strength.

My instincts told me this was the right path. After all, to change the rest of my life—to pay off $150,000 in debt, to find happiness, to get off the medication, to reclaim my self-esteem, to lose 32 pounds, to gain strength, and to rebuild my relationships—to do all of this, I knew I would first need to take control of my thoughts and my body.

During that first week I developed a plan. I began removing everything that was toxic from my life and replacing it with things that were inspiring and nourishing. I stopped hanging out with negative people and started relationships with uplifting souls who were making a positive difference. I threw out all of the toxic foods in my house and replaced them with fresh, healthful, delicious alternatives to feed my overstuffed yet undernourished body. I stopped watching mind-numbing television (canceling my cable allowed me to stick with this resolution), and started filling my brain with empowering information.

Soon I began to find myself engaged in deep, meaningful conversations with extraordinary people who were living the kind of life I wanted to live. I stopped wasting my time with worthless activities that sucked up my precious time and started recreating my body through proper nutrition and activity. Most importantly, it was during this time that I stumbled upon a secret that changed everything about my life—the way I looked, the way I felt, the way I interacted with other people. This secret gave me the keys I needed to get my life on the right track once and for all.

That secret became my new life's purpose, a philosophy to live by. I summed it up in three simple words: giving, growing, and gratitude. Or The Three Gs as I now affectionately call them. So it is with distinct pleasure that I now share these Three Gs with you:

1. **Giving.** The real rewards in life are not for those who focus on taking. No, the real rewards (happiness, self-esteem, accomplishment, and connection) are reserved for those who create value for others—in short, for the givers.

2. **Growing**. To get what I wanted out of life (and I think ultimately what we *all* want is an abundance of all that is good), I realized that it is necessary to continually grow as a person. For me, this meant that my thinking, actions, and behaviors all had to evolve. I had to align myself with what I wanted most in order to live up to my potential.

3. **Gratitude.** Happiness is rooted in the feeling of gratitude. I began feeling grateful for all of the good things in life each and every day. By focusing on the good, more good came to me, bringing joy along with it (an old friend I hadn't seen in years!).

Within 12 weeks of making the decision to change, setting a goal, following a plan, and installing this new mindset, my life was enlightened—and by this I mean that it was filled with light. That blackness I mentioned earlier? Gone!

With the help of my team I began steering my company in a completely different direction: focusing on helping, teaching, and inspiring others. As a result, I was able to pay off every last penny of the $150,000 debt I owed, avoiding the bankruptcy that seemed inevitable not too long before. (Now that, my friend, was a great day.) That very same year, I went on to buy the house of my dreams.

I created balance in my life. I started focusing on what was important (health and happiness, of course) and scheduled the moments I needed to achieve these things into my day. (I'll show you how to do this too, on page 133.) I stopped filling up on anti-anxiety medications and started dealing with stress by getting help to change my thoughts, feelings, and behaviors. I rebuilt estranged relationships by reaching out and helping others. And guess what? In return, they helped me. I started donating my time and financial resources to charities and to those in need…without expecting anything in return.

I lost the weight—32 pounds of flab—and replaced it with 10 pounds of lean, solid muscle. As a result, my confidence and energy levels went through the roof. In short, I was healthy. Not to mention happy.

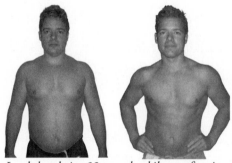

I ended up losing 32 pounds while transforming my life. I hope you'll let me help you do the same.

Although many of my goals have been reached (exceeded, even!), my transformation continues. In fact, it will continue every single day for the rest of my life. To this day, it still sometimes overwhelms me that all of this happened because of a single decision—*the decision to change.*

No matter how down and out you are, how overwhelming it all seems, you too can achieve an incredible transformation by making that first, simple decision. Stay the same or decide to change. What do *your* instincts tell you to do?

> **So what's it going to be, my friend?** Are you going to stay on your current path or make a change? Before you answer this question, before the excuses about a lack of time or money or motivation dictate your answer, think long and hard about where your current path will ultimately lead.

You have the drive inside you even if it may not seem like it just this moment. And you have the step-by-step directions, too. They're right here, in the pages that follow. The exact plan that myself and thousands of others have followed to experience a complete body and life transformation is included in this book.

If you've made the commitment to change, I welcome and congratulate you. Your new life is waiting at the end of these pages, and once you see it you'll never look back. That much I promise you.

With that in mind, I'd like to share a little bit more about how *Belly Fat Free* came to be. I initially wrote *BFF* as a way to give hope to others. I was so grateful for my new lease on life and all the opportunities the world opened up around me that I wanted to help inspire and teach others how they, too, could create a better life and realize the true version of themselves. No matter how covered up they might be by fat, sickness, and depression.

And then a big challenge emerged.

You see, after writing the first online edition of *Belly Fat Free*, I got hundreds—if not thousands—of positive e-mails and letters from good folks expressing their gratitude for the how-to information my book provided. But, even knowing what they now knew, they *still* couldn't muster up the motivation to take action.

These folks *wanted* to make a change. They weren't happy with life or with the reflection they saw staring back at them in the mirror. But they were also paralyzed by fear and a negative mindset. They needed inspiration. They needed a challenge.

So I gave them one.

And thus the Belly Fat Free Challenge was born. This Challenge is a nationwide self-improvement contest I hold each year to motivate my dear students to take the actions necessary to improve their bodies and their lives.

Every year I put up my own money, providing tens of thousands of dollars in cash and prizes. These prizes are used to inspire good folks—male and female, young and more mature—to complete a 12-week BFF Program.

> Every year I put up my own money, providing tens of thousands of dollars in cash and prizes to inspire good folks to complete a 12-week BFF Transformation Program.

When I launched this program, the feedback was immediate and overwhelming.

All told, 25,000 men and women from all over the country signed up for the Challenge. Those that followed the BFF Program saw near-immediate results in body and in spirit. Like me, they finally had hope.

I must admit, I was floored. After all, the very same people who until then had been unable to shape up for years—sometimes even decades—were suddenly achieving awe-inspiring results.

In just a few short months, men and women in their 20s, 30s, 40s, 50s, and even 60s were losing 20, 30, 40, 50, and even 100 or more pounds. What's more, they were decreasing their cholesterol levels, lowering their blood pressure, finding new relationships, rebuilding past relationships, breaking food addictions, getting off potentially harmful medications, and overcoming lifelong limitations. All while boosting their energy, self-confidence, and inner strength to sky-high levels.

It was then that I realized something I had suspected all along. In life, all of us need deadlines and motivation in order to achieve. And the more tangible, the better. Although people were certainly intrigued by the idea of a happier, healthier life, from where they stood it seemed like a near-impossible goal that would take years to achieve.

Think about it. Have you ever joined the swarms of people lined up at the post office on April 15? Have you ever seen a college library the day before final exams? Ever been shopping on December 23?

All of these examples…well, that's the power of deadlines in a nutshell. My 12-week Belly Fat Free Challenge is no different. And this, my friend, is a good thing. You may not like getting your tax return together, but you do it by April 15 because it's in your best interest. Well, the same goes for this challenge. I mean, don't get me wrong, I'd like to believe it's a more fun process than filling out your tax forms (I feel pretty confident that it is). But all you have to do is take a few simple steps, and there's a far greater prize than any tax refund waiting for you on the other side of that deadline.

Here's the gist of it. You have 12 weeks to flatten your belly (and simultaneously claim your chance at some amazing cash and prizes while you're at it). All I'm asking for is 12 weeks. That's it. And I'll be here to coach you every step of the way: through this book, through my inspirational e-mails, and live at the BellyFatFree.com interactive Web site (a very popular weight loss coaching site built to teach and inspire others how to lose belly fat for life).

Imagine where you were 12 weeks ago from today. Seriously. Think back three months from today's date. What month and day was it? Doesn't seem like that long ago, does it? My, how time flies.

> All you have to do is look three months forward, when this amazing life can be yours.

Now imagine where you would be today if you could have started this program back then. Today—this *very* day, at this *precise* moment—you would be living in a completely different body and, most likely, living a completely different life.

Right now you could be looking in the mirror and admiring your reflection—feeling proud, accomplished, and inspired. Your body could be slim and attractive. You could be happy, healthy, and living some of your best days ever, no matter your age or background.

You could be an inspirational role model to tens of thousands of people by having been named a Belly Fat Free Challenge winner. Thousands of dollars in prize winnings could already be in your pocket; cash you could use to buy a great new wardrobe, pay off your debt, or put money down on your dream home. And, speaking of dreams, you could also be proudly displaying that new beach belly of yours on one of the dream vacations just waiting to be won.

But because you didn't start the Challenge three months ago, all you have to do is look three months forward, when all of these amazing things—when this amazing *life*—can be yours. So, with all of that in mind, I have to know…what are you waiting for?

Believe me, I've gone through my own transformation. I know where you're sitting today, what you're thinking and feeling, and I can say with total conviction that there will *never* be a more perfect time to begin transforming your life than right this second.

The very fact that you have this book in your hands is not an accident. In life, really, there are no accidents. Everything has a purpose. We've met for a reason. And that reason is to help you achieve the body and life you truly deserve. My goal is to see you accomplish exactly that.

I've been where you are. I've felt unhappy, uncertain, skeptical, and confused. I've planted my feet down, refusing to change my own life simply because it sounded like too much work, or took up too much time, or sounded too good to be true. But take it from me, you have to move past all of the excuses...because that's all they are. No matter what or how many reservations you have, I want you to know that *I* believe in your ability to change and transform. I believe in you, even if you don't yet believe in yourself. And I'm here to help guide you over to that brighter path.

So, if you are sick and tired of being out of control, overweight, and low on confidence; if you acknowledge that this may truly be the single perfect moment to begin living up to your true potential, then I encourage you to accept my challenge and continue on the path you've already begun.

And now, my friend, we're in it together.

BFF Assignment #1 ☐
Help Me Help You

As your Belly Fat Free Coach, throughout this book I'll be asking you to take part in a variety of assignments that will help move you toward your ultimate transformation. With that in mind, here's your very first assignment.

It's simple. Just visit BellyFatFree.com and sign up for this year's BFF Challenge. There are thousands of dollars in cash and prizes up for grabs for those who take action and make the most inspiring transformations. Plus, BellyFatFree.com is a community thousands of members strong. Everyone is in it together, ready to encourage and motivate you when you need it most.

Who knows? Maybe your story will be the next one to inspire others to recreate their life as well. Because that, my friend, is what life is all about—helping and encouraging others.

BFF Success Story
Gail: An Artist Sculpts a New Body

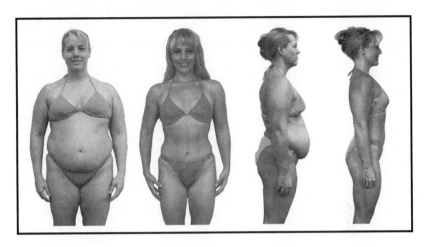

Gail Gosselin, a 40-year-old artist and waitress, lost 53 pounds in the Belly Fat Free Challenge. That in and of itself is impressive. But get this: Gail pulled this off while working at an Italian restaurant.

Gail had spent most of her life overweight. Fat. Miserable. Growing up, the kids in school were relentlessly mean. By the time she got into high school, a bout with acne made everything even worse. The other kids began to call her "Walking Ugly."

Gail so badly wanted to date like everyone else. But think back to your high school and you can imagine that none of the boys wanted to be caught dead going out with Walking Ugly. So she never went out on dates, missing out on rites of passage like her high school prom along the way.

It's not surprising that before long it got to the point where Gail suffered from low energy, very low self-esteem, even depression because of all the extra fat she was carrying around. So she started to abuse her body even more—she developed eating disorders. For decades Gail starved and binged, sometimes losing belly fat but always gaining it back in the end because she never learned how to lose weight correctly…and keep it off for good. "Everything in my life felt like a struggle," Gail remembers. "I had no energy."

When she signed up for the BFF Challenge, Gail didn't keep it a secret. In fact, she did quite the opposite. She told her friends and co-workers about it and asked them to lend their support. "There's no way anyone I worked with would let me cheat," she recalls, laughing. "They all wanted to see me win."

According to Gail, after all those years of taunting and depression, sadness and pain, in the end losing the weight was surprisingly simple. "I focused my mind on my goals and then everything seemed to just fall into place."

All told, Gail lost 53 pounds, 47 inches of fat, and dropped seven dress sizes. (Just look at how her belly disappeared!) But that's not all. When she traded fat for lean muscle, Gail *felt* better too. "My energy levels have increased dramatically and the backaches and leg cramps I was suffering from due to the excess weight have disappeared, as well as a lot of unsightly cellulite. I feel healthy, I look healthy, and I am beyond happy.

"I don't feel like I'm even the same person as I was before following Belly Fat Free and starting the Challenge," she enthuses. "I feel as though I've freed myself from the mental prison of going through the motions of life on autopilot. I am so much more outgoing now, and things don't get me down as easily as they did before. I joke around a lot more too, because I'm not self-conscious about drawing attention to myself. I am so full of confidence and energy that I not only look different, but I act different too."

"I've completely changed my way of thinking. I make workout dates instead of lunch dates and I organize gym 'field trips' with my co-workers and art studio mates. I feel as though I've climbed to the top of a mountain and, as I stood on the highest peak and looked down, I realized that I had virtually the whole world at my feet. I can accomplish anything I set my mind to. I feel stronger inside and out, and my newfound confidence has helped me believe in myself again. Now I can help others work at achieving their weight loss goals as well, and that feels really good."

CHAPTER 3

Your Thoughts Control Your Weight

Now before we get into the nuts and bolts of the BFF Program, I have an important question. When the going gets tough, are you a sinker or a swimmer?

I'm betting you're a swimmer...otherwise you wouldn't be with me today. What I mean by this is when the going gets tough, you're probably not the type to give up and give in. For you, sinking probably isn't even an option.

I've never been a sinker. I used to be a swimmer, but not anymore. You see, nowadays, I try not to even get in the water. Instead I simply build a bridge.

Let me explain. When the going gets tough—which it *always* does at some point—a sinker will...well, sink. Conversely, a swimmer will fight tooth and nail to keep her head above water. Now a *bridge builder*, on the other hand, will anticipate obstacles and plan for future events before they happen so that she doesn't set foot in the water—not even a toe—or have to work extremely hard for victory.

With that in mind, we've already discussed the Challenge at hand. I'm asking you, or better yet, *challenging* you, to take the next 12 weeks to get into the best shape of your life.

Now the majority of people will hear about the Challenge and do nothing. They'll sink. Others will take the Challenge on immediately (without planning) and plunge head first into the rapids, fighting like crazy against the tide (and many times against themselves) in their attempts at transformation.

But it's been my experience that only a select few will first take the time to build the bridge necessary for success. Building a bridge may sound difficult but, in fact, it's really not hard work at all…it's *smart* work. And the greatest thing is, I've already built it for you.

All you need to do is apply a few strategies to your life and simply stroll along your bridge—over the icy cold rapids swirling below, where all the sinkers and swimmers will be bobbing like apples. (But I hope you will take the time to "fish out" those in need. I know that's what I'll be doing.)

With that in mind, here are my tried and true techniques for progressing forward—*rapidly*—toward your BFF dreams and goals. Make no mistake, this is your bridge to a brighter future. It's your bridge over troubled waters, which will safely transport you from desperation to inspiration. The more closely you follow these instructions, the sturdier your bridge will be. But if you don't follow this path, chances are you will slip and fall. (But I will do my best to pull you to safety if you do, so don't be afraid to try.)

Do you want to know my very best secret to transforming your body—a seven-minute secret that will work wonders for you even if you choose to do nothing else mentioned in this chapter?

Well, wait no longer, my secret is here.

The BFF Confidence Booster™

Real and lasting change starts on the inside. The very first step to success of any variety is fueling your mind with positive thoughts, images, and emotions. You've got to understand that pain *will* persist if you continue on your present path. You can, however, decide to let pleasure and improvement prevail by taking a different path.

In my experience, the number one reason most people never fully gain control over their bodies (which is done by losing weight and keeping it off) is because they don't have the confidence to do so. Their self-esteem is injured…especially if they've tried and failed to lose weight multiple times in the past.

Coupled with the fact that society has a real knack for sucking the potential and confidence right on out of us, this can be a real killer. The media plays a big role by setting unrealistic examples about what is attractive through movie, magazine, and TV stars. Many men and women then develop inadequate feelings, comparing themselves to these unattainable examples.

Others try to emulate the current trend of "what is attractive," which almost always involves losing weight and getting in better shape. But, the **big** problem is they go about this in the wrong way, following gimmicky diet plans and overnight miracle products. When they don't see results, their belief and confidence in themselves starts to deteriorate.

What's more, since childhood many of us have been constantly reminded of our imperfections and what we are *not*; too often the negative rather than positive is highlighted. As a result, many people don't feel they deserve the best in life.

I'm sure you can recall many times in your life when in not so many words (or maybe in big, loud words), you were told you weren't smart enough, too young or too old, not from the right economic background, the wrong ethnicity, not disciplined enough, not strong enough, too short or too tall, not attractive enough, and so on. (Do you remember any of these times?)

Believe me, friend, after a while this type of negative programming becomes ingrained into your thoughts and actions. Pretty soon you may think that you don't deserve to have an abundance of all that is good in life, or that you will never achieve anything worthwhile.

Well, I'm here to tell you loud and clear that's all a bunch of baloney. You *do* deserve to be *extraordinary* and to have an abundant, amazing life. What's more, you can achieve something inspiring—like creating your own slim body—no matter what anyone says. No matter how many times you've failed in the past. (That's assuming you go about it the right way this time, of course.)

By now you're probably thinking this sounds all fine and dandy, but how do you actually do this—how do you build certainty and confidence? Great question. My answer is the BFF Confidence Booster™.

Reprogram Your Mind to Transform Your Body

Every day I get e-mails and see journal and forum posts at BellyFatFree.com from hundreds of good folks who want to know, "How can I increase my self-esteem and self-confidence?" I love this question because it's one of the best, most important questions anyone could ever ask. After all, the answer is the secret to transforming your body. Besides, who couldn't use more confidence in his or her life?

You see, it's been my observation that the most successful people in the world—those who have success in *all* areas of life— are extremely confident people. Believe me, there is one thing all of the top athletes, business people, leaders, and philanthropists from our history have in common, and that's a high level of confidence. But not all of them started with it.

I want you to know that confidence can be developed. You can grow it, just like a muscle. You can transform it, just like you can transform your body. Speaking of transforming your body, it's no secret that recreating your body means you must first remove the negative (too much "bad" food and inactivity) and replace it with the positive (good foods and activity). Your confidence is no different. To transform it, you must remove the negative—self-defeating thoughts, feelings, and attitudes—and focus on the positive.

The fact is, your confidence needs nourishment every single day. It's just like your body. If you don't nourish your body, you get sick. If you don't nourish your confidence you become uncertain, sad, stressed, and frustrated. (And many people have been living in this state of mind for years—sometimes decades.)

It's such a shame that millions of people are walking around with a "disease" called low self-confidence (or low self-esteem). And truth be told, it may not be rock-bottom low, but it's low enough to keep them from their real potential and from achieving what they really want out of life.

Let's say, for example, you have a confidence level of a six (on a scale of one to 10 with 10 being the highest), but you're trying to accomplish a goal that requires a confidence level of nine. Do you see the problem here? Your confidence won't be in sync with your goal and, nine times out of 10, you will fail. Or you'll reach your goal only to revert back to status quo because your self-esteem and your goal weren't in alignment.

Think about this: I've discovered that most people perform to a level that is equal to their confidence level. High confidence equals high performance. Low confidence equals low performance. *More than that, most people create a life that is equal to their confidence level as well.* (Please reread that sentence and think about it carefully. What kind of life has your confidence allowed you to create so far?)

> I've discovered that most people perform to a level that is equal to their confidence level.

Let's try looking at it this way.

On a scale from one to 10 (again with 10 being the highest), what is your current overall confidence level? Be honest. Okay. Now, on that same scale, how would you rate your happiness with your life overall?

I bet these two numbers are very close. You can't be happier than your self-esteem allows you to be. Your confidence represents a ceiling for everything else in your life. Let me now ask you how successful you feel in life, using the same scale? (And please note, I'm not asking how you compare against others, but how you *feel*.) I bet it's near the same level at which you perceive your confidence and happiness to be. What level are most of your relationships? See what I'm getting at? It's very difficult to outperform your confidence levels in any area of life.

We all have ceilings—self-imposed barriers that control everything we're able to do. How we feel about ourselves. How happy we are. How much we can accomplish in life. What we feel we deserve. The question now becomes this: How can you increase your confidence and break through those mental barriers so you can transform your body and live a happier life? After all, to achieve the goal of transforming your body in as little as 12 weeks, you're going to need to turbo charge your confidence levels…and fast.

This is where my BFF Confidence Booster comes into play. And here's the first rule: **You have to make your confidence a top priority.** You must protect it, nourish it, and celebrate it. Why? Because from what I've seen, people with low confidence levels (a six or below) tend to put themselves last on the list after everyone else (especially family). Many times they aren't even *on* the list.

And more times than not, people with low confidence are also rooted in history. By this I mean they tend to focus more on the past—or just getting by now in the present—than on creating an incredible future. But remember, the past is nothing more than a memory in your mind. It can be erased and recorded over. Instead of letting negative past events play over and over in your mind, destroying your valuable confidence in the process, you can scratch that record and start playing a new, empowering one.

How? Begin by changing your thoughts and your focus on a day-to-day basis. This will change how you feel and what you do in life—your daily actions. It will lead you toward your goals. In a sense, it will reprogram you from the inside out.

Here's an example. A year ago, a woman named Emily came to me for help. She had gotten married young and had two children. Unfortunately, her husband turned out to be a very emotionally abusive man. After years of abuse, he left Emily and their kids for another woman and started a new family with her. As you can imagine, Emily's already fragile self-esteem plummeted.

Emily had gained a lot of weight during her roller coaster marriage, but during the divorce and immediately after she started feeding her emotions even more and gained an additional 40 pounds (she was 75 pounds overweight in total). This only caused her self-esteem to fall further.

When I met Emily the first thing I asked her was, "On a scale of one to 10, with 10 being the highest, how would you rate your confidence level?" Emily answered, "Two." I knew this meant her overall happiness in life was near a two as well. (This is a very dangerous level, by the way. There isn't much further to fall.)

Because Emily's self-esteem was so low, she had stopped caring for herself and made her children her entire life. What's more, she was so afraid her children would leave her to go live with their father that she gave in to their every whim—which included having junk food at nearly every meal—causing her children to become overweight and insecure as well.

It had been two years since the divorce and Emily still lacked the self-esteem to date. She passed up job opportunities and her finances were in big trouble—she lived hand to mouth with each paycheck, borrowing money from relatives just to get by.

Emily couldn't escape her past and, until we met, she refused to look at her future. She lacked the self-esteem to realize that she really *did* have the power to create the kind of life she wanted… and, more than that, the kind of life she deserved. Emily came to me for weight loss advice, but I knew her confidence level wouldn't allow her to be successful. Instead we needed to first focus on increasing her confidence. We needed to transform her from the inside out. Outside-in approaches (like exercise and healthy eating) only work if you have a high enough self-esteem to follow through and make them stick in the long run. (I estimate that 90 percent of dieters don't have this confidence level to begin with, so they fail.)

To help boost Emily's confidence, I began by giving her a simple assignment: On a piece of paper, I had her write down five things in her life she was really grateful for. This wasn't easy for Emily because she was used to focusing on what she *didn't* like about her life. But I'm here to tell you that in life you end up getting what you think about the most. If you constantly put yourself down and remind yourself of what you aren't or of everything that is wrong, you get more of exactly that.

In my own life, I've discovered that thoughts act just like a magnet, drawing whatever you focus on most toward you. Scientists have been studying thoughts for decades, and they really do create measurable energy. Have you ever heard of the power of prayer? Well, prayers are nothing more than thoughts. Science has proven that thoughts can create things. They also control your emotions. That's why it's so important to be positive even if you don't really believe your positive thoughts in the beginning. You will—it just takes a little practice.

> I've discovered that thoughts act just like a magnet, drawing whatever you focus on most toward you.

If you think and feel great, you get more of that. If you think and feel bad…well, you get more of that, too. (I'm not suggesting you ignore that which is bad, simply that you fix it and move forward, while focusing on the good things in your life—and the good lessons you've learned from any mistakes.)

The power of positive thinking…you can't escape it. But you *can* use it to your advantage. It's why the rich get richer and the poor get poorer. It's why the healthy stay healthy and the sick get sicker. It's why the happy get happier and the depressed get more depressed. And, believe it or not, you have control over most of this simply by what you focus on.

Do you think what I'm saying is all a bunch of mumbo-jumbo? If so, don't worry. I'm not about to bring out a crystal ball and start chanting. But make no mistake, your thoughts are extremely powerful. Thoughts have the power to create success or failure, happiness or sadness, an extraordinary life or an ordinary life.

What I'm talking about here is nothing new. High achievers have been using the power of positive thought for years. People like Oprah Winfrey, Michael Jordan, Bill Gates, Hillary Clinton, Mother Teresa, Martin Luther King Jr., and Presidents like Ronald Reagan and Barack Obama. Even great scientists, artists, and philosophers throughout history have written extensively about the power of thought (Einstein, Plato, Newton, Carnegie, Beethoven, and Shakespeare, just to name a few).

This, my friend, is the great secret of life. You're already using the power of thought to attract things into your life, so why not harness the power of positive thinking to attract whatever it is that you want most. Perhaps a new flat belly, better finances, more happiness?

You Get What You Focus on Most

Like all of us, Emily was attracting that which she focused on most. She focused on her failed marriage. She constantly thought about why she wasn't good enough. She focused on how unattractive she felt because of her weight. She focused on how much of a failure she felt like in her career and as a mother. She focused on not living up to her potential. And she focused on her negative past and current unhappiness. Well, guess what? That is exactly what she got more of.

After explaining all of this to me, Emily still couldn't think of much she was grateful for. So I helped her change her physical and mental state. Here is what I said to her: "Emily, I want you to close your eyes and imagine a time in your life where you felt great about yourself. Got it? Okay, now I want you to breathe the way you were breathing then. Good. Now I want you to take on the posture you had then. Now I want you to smile the way you smiled then and talk the way you talked then. And walk the way you walked then. Excellent."

By doing this we changed Emily's physical state, which in turn changed how she was feeling emotionally. She stopped slouching in her chair. She sat up straight. She began to breathe deeply. Heck, you could practically see her confidence rising as she did this assignment. I then once again asked Emily what her confidence level felt like. This time she said, "A six." Remember, just a few minutes earlier she was at a two.

> **Tip:** You can use these same techniques to change your mood any time you wish. Your mind will follow your body's example. Research studies have proven this when scientists had depressed patients do nothing but smile for 30 minutes at a time. Doing this worked better than antidepressant medication in many cases.

Now that Emily was feeling better she was finally able to write down five things she was grateful for. Here is what she wrote:

1. I am grateful for the laughter in my life.

2. I am grateful for the money I make at work.

3. I am grateful for the health of my family and friends.

4. I am grateful for my ability to make the decision to change my life.

5. I am grateful for being an attentive mother who is involved with and loves her children.

Well, guess what? After this little assignment Emily had a smile on her face. She actually felt somewhat okay about herself for the first time in a long time. Why? Because it's impossible to feel sad, frustrated, scared, or anxious when you're feeling grateful. (It's true. Try this the next time you want to change your emotional state: Start thinking about everything in your life that you are really grateful for. Talk about these things out loud with passion and really feel the powerful emotions they evoke.)

Next I had Emily write down five specific things she admired most about herself. Here is what she wrote:

1. I love my smile.

2. I love the way I play with my children.

3. I love my curly hair.

4. I love the way I compliment people and make them feel better.

5. I love my intelligence and my ability to get things done.

Through this assignment Emily began to nourish her confidence. Her self-esteem had been deprived for so long that this was like giving water to a near-dead plant—she soaked up the nourishment quickly, and it began to show.

Now come closer; I want to whisper an important secret to you. Ready? Here it is: In life, you can't count on other people to build your self-esteem for you. Otherwise you'll be waiting forever. Your self-esteem represents your heart and soul. It's the energy of life. It is the most important thing you will ever possess. Your self-esteem even impacts your health. It truly is a gift. And it's up to *you* to protect and build it every single day. No matter what.

(By the way, do you want to know what I think the purpose of life is? I think our purpose in life is to follow our bliss—to do that which makes us most happy in the long run—to build our self-love and let that spill out to those around us, helping them in the process. I think it is as simple...and as wonderful...as that.)

Moving Forward with Emily

Next, I asked Emily to write down five things she had done in the past, things she hadn't thought she was capable of doing at the time or that she thought would be very difficult.

She wrote:

1. I got the starring role in a high school play and we received three standing ovations.

2. I graduated from college with a 3.2 grade point average.

3. I've kept a job for 10 years when a lot of other employees were laid off.

4. I have raised two respectable children as a single mother.

5. I have headed up fundraising events at my church, raising more than $5,000 to help the less fortunate.

This assignment fed Emily's self-confidence even more and helped remind her that she has accomplished a lot of difficult tasks in the past—tasks that may have seemed impossible at the time—and it reminded her that she could use this same inner strength to transform her body as well.

Next I asked Emily a very important question: "Over the next 12 weeks, what five specific things have to happen for you to feel thrilled with your results in life?" Here's the catch: I added that she had to write her response as though she *already* accomplished these goals. Emily wrote these 12-week goals:

1. I have lost 20 pounds of body fat.

2. I have gained four pounds of muscle tone and doubled my physical strength.

3. I have increased my daily confidence level from a two to an eight.

4. I have started dating again and am dating only quality men.

5. Each of my children has lost 10 pounds because I have taught them what I've learned about taking care of myself.

I then had Emily read these five 12-week goals out loud with passion and asked her to imagine what it would look like and feel like to have this kind of success. By this time, Emily was smiling from ear to ear. She felt hope—one of the most powerful emotions—because she was finally able to see a brighter, happier future.

> Hope is one of the most powerful emotions.

I asked Emily what word described how she felt right now. She said, "Success." I asked her to remember that word, and told her that any time she felt bad and wanted to feel good, all she needed to do was to say or think the word "success" and all of these wonderful emotions would come flooding back to her. (That's an important tip, by the way. I hope you'll try this technique, too.)

Next I asked Emily this question: "In order for you to achieve these five goals over the next 12 weeks, what five characteristics will you need to possess in order to ensure your success?" My friend, please reread that question again. It's a very powerful one. The reality is, in order to accomplish great things, you first have to realize the "success characteristics" a person must have to achieve them.

For example, if you have the goal of tripling your income over the next year but you sleep 18 hours a day and spend the other six hours watching TV, you obviously aren't the type of person who has yet developed the characteristics to achieve this goal. Similarly, if your goal is to lose 20 pounds in 12 weeks but you're constantly eating junk food, you're not planning, you're skipping workouts, you're not building your self-esteem, and you're not making your goal a priority, it's very clear that you're not going to be successful.

I can tell you this with complete certainty: In order to get what you want in life, you must become the type of person who can attract these good things to you.

With that in mind, Emily's "to be" goals, stated as though she already possessed them, were:

1. I am a dedicated person who plans and keeps track of my progress.

2. I am a diligent person who consistently follows through on my plan.

3. I am a persistent person who doesn't give up even when challenges arise. I am a person who focuses on finding solutions, not problems.

4. I am a happy person who nourishes my confidence daily, knowing that I'll then have more energy to give to others.

5. I am an inspiring person who teaches others to live a healthy, happy life.

I then had Emily read each of these success characteristics out loud, with passion, while imagining a situation where she was performing each of these five characteristics and enjoying every moment of it. (For example, for number two she imagined herself happily exercising and eating healthy, delicious foods—all part of her Belly Fat Free plan.)

Make no mistake, these are characteristics that everyone must develop in order to accomplish any worthy goal. (And I'm here to help you every step of the way.)

Recipe for Success

The last assignment I gave Emily is the most important of all. I asked her to spend just seven minutes a day feeding her self-confidence, as we had just done. Specifically, I asked her to begin by reflecting on and *feeling* what she was most grateful for in her life. (Remember, life brings you what you focus on most. If you're grateful for what you currently have, you get more of what you're grateful for.)

Next I asked her to spend a moment thinking about what she liked best about herself, reminding her again to change her physical state—her posture and her breathing—to help put her in a confident state.

I then asked Emily to imagine what it felt like to have achieved her 12-week goals. (It's important to imagine them as if they have already happened. On a subconscious level, your mind can't tell the difference between something you imagine to be real, versus reality…and it will work to bring your thoughts into reality.) To help with this I told Emily to create a *mental movie* complete with inspiring music that displayed what her body would look like after 12 weeks, how she felt in this new body, how she felt with "level-eight" confidence, and what it was like to see her children 10 pounds lighter, happier, and healthier.

I asked her to imagine what it was like to shop for new clothes in her new body. I instructed her to see people smiling at her and to hear their compliments. I reminded her to visualize herself looking in the mirror and loving her reflection. I asked her to see a life that was so enticing she felt compelled to do what it took to have it.

Finally, I had Emily imagine what it felt like to be the person she needed to be in order to achieve her goals. I asked her to imagine herself following a good eating and exercise program, being consistent, feeling great, staying on course, avoiding junk food, putting herself first, accomplishing goals, building her confidence, inspiring others, and feeling joyous throughout the entire process.

I asked her to create this mental movie—to see it and feel it—every day during her down time. When she was getting ready for work in the morning, when she took her dog for a walk, while driving to work, during a break, driving home, during TV commercials, or just before bed.

> **Tip:** I highly recommend making a seven-minute audio recording with a little digital recorder to guide you through your mental movie. Maybe your movie is about an underdog and everything she went through to come out a champion at the end of the movie. After all, this is one of Hollywood's favorite plots, and it could very well become the story of your life!

I next asked Emily to put up "visual reminders," like a picture of herself when she was at her ideal weight or a picture of someone else's body she wanted to emulate (with a similar body type) to remind her of her body transformation goal and how she would feel every time she took a step toward achieving it. (I had her put these visual reminders on her bathroom mirror, refrigerator, and on her computer so she'd see them throughout the day.)

I even instructed Emily to feel what it would feel like to have her dream body every time she handled her set of keys (which was about eight times a day). Not only did this assignment help boost Emily's confidence, it also gave her mind a crystal-clear goal to focus on and to draw toward her.

Now I'm giving this very same assignment to you.

BFF Assignment #2 ☐
Practice the Belly Fat Free
Confidence Booster

If you're tired of living a so-so life, if you're sick and tired of being sick and tired, if you're finally ready to end the excuses and to start living up to your full potential, then I want you to take the first step toward transforming your life right now. Turn to page 47 and carefully fill out the Belly Fat Free Confidence Booster form. Remember, this will be an invaluable tool throughout the course of your 12-week transformation, so be sure to answer as honestly and accurately as possible.

Seven Minutes a Day

Now that you have this vital information, the key is to consistently use it for just seven minutes to build your confidence levels—your inner strength and desire—each and every day.

To recap, for seven minutes once every day you'll want to:

1. Remind yourself about five things you are currently grateful for. (Start by saying or thinking, "I am grateful for…".)

2. Say (out loud) five things you admire most about yourself. (Be sure to *feel* the positive feelings while you're doing this. For most people, a big smile will appear on their faces.)

3. Think about five things you've already accomplished in life and how great you felt after achieving them.

4. Think about your five 12-week transformation goals as if you've already achieved them. Focus on the feeling of reaching your goals and how having a new and improved body is going to affect all areas of your life in a positive way. Create a mental movie with you as the star. Maybe you want to see yourself celebrating with the other Belly Fat Free Challenge Champions and me.

5. Think about and *feel* the Five Success Characteristics you've added into your life. (Hint: See yourself planning; exercising; eating healthy, tasty foods every three hours; overcoming challenges; tracking your progress; nourishing your confidence; and celebrating your results.)

That's how simple it is to completely transform your confidence levels, which will in turn allow you to accomplish your dreams and goals.

When I first started doing this technique, I had a hard time with it. My mind would wander and it was hard for me to stay on track. Then I made an audio recording (with a little Olympus digital recorder I got at BestBuy.com for $39) that walked me through each of the five steps and my answers to the questions. All I did was close my eyes, put on my headphones, and follow along in my mind. This may work well for you, too.

Believe me, folks, this BFF Confidence Booster is vital to your success with this program, or any other program, for that matter. Come to think of it, it's critical to having a successful, happy life in general.

The Key Is to Make It Fun and Exciting... Something You Love Doing

You should look forward to doing this mindset exercise each day. For me, it releases these amazing feelings of confidence, clarity, connection, purpose, accomplishment, and joy. I encourage you to use it daily. Those that do are the type of people who will succeed at recreating their bodies and living happy and healthy lives. Those that won't, aren't.

Remember, you can't outperform your confidence level. If you don't have the confidence (or self-esteem) necessary to accomplish a goal, either it won't happen, it will be very difficult, or the results won't last. You may see results for a few weeks, but they will quickly end or you'll sabotage your efforts. (Has this ever happened to you during a past weight loss attempt? Now you know why. You must transform your confidence in order to transform your body.)

But now, finally, there is hope because when you follow the BFF Confidence Booster for just seven minutes a day...

I Can Promise You This:

✔ You will replace bad habits with empowering ones.

✔ You will begin to automatically crave the taste of healthier foods and you'll feel full and satisfied with less food.

✔ You will develop positive addictions like moving your body and feeling great.

✔ You will have greater control over your thoughts and emotions, and great things will be attracted into your life.

✔ You will successfully transform your body faster and easier than you ever thought possible.

✔ You will build stronger relationships.

✔ You will create a happy, beautiful life and live up to your true potential.

This I know for sure.

Keep Promises to Yourself

Finally, remember that it is imperative to do what you tell yourself you will do and keep the promises you make to yourself. I can't stress this enough. Would you trust a friend who constantly lied to you? Of course not. But sadly, millions of people in this world make promises to themselves and fail to follow through. Soon they begin to distrust themselves, which is a very bad thing.

Let me ask you: Where do you think anxiety, insecurity, fear, and uncertainty come from? Do you think not keeping self-promises may cause some of these emotions? Let me assure you, it does.

When you don't honor self-promises, you start to erode your treasured self-confidence. If you lie to yourself your self-esteem pays the price—meaning your life pays the price. The good news is to build confidence you simply need to follow through and do what you say you're going to do. It will make all the difference in the world. And it all begins by following through with the BFF Confidence Booster once a day. In fact, that's what Emily started doing. She started keeping her self-promise to follow this program. (Speaking of, I bet you're wondering what happened to Emily.)

Emily's Transformation

Emily followed the five steps of the BFF Confidence Booster every day, even on those days when she just had a minute or two to spare. By doing this she completely transformed her confidence levels. She also followed the eating, activity, and supplement program I will outline in upcoming chapters. At the end of 12 weeks we met again to review her progress. Here are her accomplishments:

1. She lost 26 pounds of body fat (her goal was 20 pounds). Her cholesterol also decreased from 243 to 187.

2. She gained five pounds of muscle and more than doubled the weight she was using for all of her core resistance exercises (her goal was to add four pounds of muscle and double her strength).

3. Her new perceived confidence level was an eight (her goal was an eight).

4. She met a quality man from her church whom she was dating exclusively—and happily, I might add (beginning to date quality men was one of her goals).

5. She taught a new way of thinking and a new healthy lifestyle to both of her children, who lost a combined 18 pounds while increasing their grades at school (her goal was to help her two children lose 10 pounds each).

Nearly every one of Emily's 12-week goals came true because she used the power of her own mind—her own thoughts and feelings—to increase her confidence and to take action to become the person she needed to become in order to be successful.

And, as you already know, Emily is not the only one to accomplish goals like these, nor will she be the last. This book is filled with extraordinary, real-life success stories from amazing people who have learned how to harness the power of their own minds, to help them transform all areas of their lives.

If you haven't already, I encourage you to answer the questions above and make your own BFF Confidence Booster recording to listen to during the day. Believe me, this will be your bridge over troubled waters. It will lead you from where you are now to where you want to be in 12 weeks.

That is my promise to you.

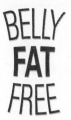
BELLY FAT FREE

BFF Confidence Booster™

Date:	Goal Weight:	Days To Deadline:

What are you grateful for today?

1. _____
2. _____
3. _____
4. _____
5. _____

What do you admire most about yourself?

1. _____
2. _____
3. _____
4. _____
5. _____

What are your biggest achievements so far in life?

1. _____
2. _____
3. _____
4. _____
5. _____

Before your 12-week deadline, what five things must occur for you to feel successful?

1. _____
2. _____
3. _____
4. _____
5. _____

What five habits will you need to develop to reach your goals?

1. _____
2. _____
3. _____
4. _____
5. _____

Notes: _____

_____

Your Thoughts Control Your Weight   47

BFF Success Story
Marcia: Defying Time With a Slimmer, Stronger, Healthier Body

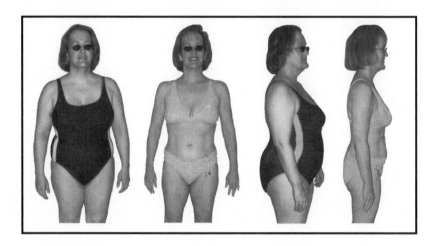

Marcia needed a new outfit to wear to a celebratory dinner for her daughter's high school graduation. But her anticipated joy soon turned to frustration and sadness. She was looking for a nice pair of black slacks. Not too difficult, right? One wouldn't think so, but when Marcia tried on several pairs in her usual size 14, she couldn't zip them up. Not even when she held in her breath. Finally, after foraging through racks and racks of clothes, Marcia managed to find one tight size 16 she could squeeze into—in white. As she sucked in her stomach and zipped up the slacks she said to herself, "Well, I guess I won't be eating much tonight."

The graduation itself was magnificent and all the families snapped photographs of the event. Marcia remembers, "When I looked at our photograph, I saw our daughter wearing her cap and gown and her father and I standing beside her. I was there smiling for the picture, but inside I was so embarrassed and so ashamed of the way I looked. I could have cried." That was Marcia's defining moment, the moment when she knew she could no longer go on as she was. She had to do something about her weight.

There were also other important reasons for Marcia to transform her body. Her doctor had been after her to drop some weight, saying it would help lessen the migraine headaches Marcia had been suffering from for years. She was on prescription medication and thought it would be great to get rid of the expensive bill. High cholesterol was also an issue. Each time she went to the doctor, her cholesterol was up a little more. Because both her mom and dad suffered from high cholesterol, Marcia was concerned about heart disease.

Although Marcia knew she had to lose weight, the timing was daunting. "My biggest beef is that losing weight is harder for women like me who are going through menopause. We've got issues related to our hormones. I started studying and I learned that our hormones affect so much of what goes on in our bodies. So, yes, my body was fighting me. But I decided to fight back."

Changing hormones were not Marcia's only battle. One day while she was gardening, dark, jagged lines shot into her vision. Then a couple days later, a black patch obstructed some of her view. The retina in Marcia's right eye detached, and she was rushed into surgery. "At first, I was feeling pretty darn sorry for myself. Mostly, I was angry with myself for letting all that weight pile up. Now with the eye surgery, I had yet another excuse not to exercise. But then I said to myself, 'Well, I'm still here. What can I do?' I chose to focus on transforming my body."

Marcia took the leap and signed up for the BFF Challenge. She got a high-tech scale that measures fitness level or *metabolic age*. Although Marcia's real age was 48, her metabolic age was more than 50. That was not good.

Marcia says her biggest key to success was implementing the entire program. She realized she couldn't expect the program to work for her if she didn't do it all. Well, Marcia's hard work paid off. **Despite the many obstacles she faced, Marcia lost 52 pounds, 37 inches, and brought her BMI down from 31.8 (obese) to a healthy 23.2.** As if all that wasn't enough, Marcia's cholesterol went down from 248 to 182, her migraines are fewer and further between, and her metabolic age now has this 48-year-old registering at 32 years of age.

"What's most important is that I'm confident I'm going to live longer, with a high quality of life, and that works just fine for me and my family," Marcia says. And what about those tight size 16 white slacks—the ones she bought for her daughter's high school graduation? She now slides into a size eight with no problem.

CHAPTER 4

The Obesity Conspiracy Exposed

There's a big fat cover up they don't want you to know about. What am I talking about?

The Great American Obesity Conspiracy. And, as is the case with all conspiracies, all you have to do to find the culprits is follow the money.

So who exactly is profiting from you and your loved ones gaining belly fat, losing confidence, becoming sick (or worse), and *staying* that way? That's a darn good question. Here are the top villains:

1. **Giant food manufacturers .** Some of the greedy corporate executives who run these publicly traded companies habitually demand that addictive obesity additives be added into foods and beverages that line our grocery store shelves. These (mostly) man-made chemicals can lead to severe food addictions, causing people to eat more and more (and, subsequently, *buy* more and more) while unsavory food giants haul in record profits.

2. **The big, bad pharmaceutical giants and the medical industry.** Keep in mind that the drug companies don't make profits by helping you become slim and healthy. On the contrary, their big profits come from force feeding you and your family dozens of medications to control such weight-related conditions as high blood pressure, depression, certain cancers, high cholesterol, anxiety, heartburn, insomnia, low energy, erectile dysfunction, gout, and diabetes…just to name a few. The goal of these companies is to make you a pill-popping client for life.

   Even more terrifying is the fact that pharmaceutical giants virtually own doctors. They control most of the curriculum in medical schools as well as the continuing education classes doctors are required to take.

   Unfortunately, this means doctors are learning to push a pill or a procedure rather than getting to the root of the problem, which in many cases revolves around nutritional issues. Doctors today should keep in mind what the Greek physician and father of medicine, Hippocrates, said more than 2,000 years ago: "Let medicine be our food, and food be our medicine." (Read more about how the medical and pharmaceutical companies are conspiring to hurt your health in Chapter 5.)

3. **Rip-off weight loss companies.** The majority of weight loss gadgets, gizmos, and diet plans advertised on television, radio, and in magazines simply don't work…and if they do, most people can't follow them for long.

   In this chapter we'll concentrate on food manufacturers, and I'll let you in on important information you need to know about what they're putting in your food and what you can do to break the obesity additive cycle. Read on to find out about how all of this contributes to America's big fat problem.

Giant Food Manufacturers

It all started when I began interviewing many of the world's *top* scientists and doctors to find out why my dear students and I couldn't lose belly fat. I was shocked to hear of the new research on food additives and preservatives (chemicals) that are quietly being added to our foods.

It turns out that piles of new research studies—from the top universities—show that these chemicals are making us sick, fat, and *addicted* for life. This way we keep eating and eating without ever getting full and satisfied, while *seedy* food manufacturers make record profits year after year. (Do you ever have uncontrollable cravings?)

> Many of the chemicals all too commonly found in today's foods can be just as addictive as alcohol, cigarettes, and even various street drugs.

Did you know that most of the tens of thousands of food items that are lining our grocery store shelves are made and controlled by only four or five GIANT, multinational food corporations that have only *one* goal in mind—to make more and more money? It's true. (Watch the movie Food Inc. for complete details.)

These mammoth food giants' primary goal isn't to create healthy food or to help America stay slim—their actions are controlled by Wall Street and greedy CEOs and "money men" secretly scheming and plotting behind closed doors.

The reality is that these food chemists create "Frankenstein foods" within these huge, robotic, assembly-line factories. Here they dump all kinds of man-made preservatives, additives, and chemicals into the recipes for our favorite meals and snacks—in just the right amounts—so these "fake foods" can sit on grocery

The Obesity Conspiracy Exposed

53

store shelves for months, years, and even decades without going bad.

WARNING: A side effect of some of these food additives is that they can change our brain chemistry, causing us to become addicted and gain body fat.

Then they slap a label on the food product showing a wholesome family farm and spend billions of dollars advertising the food as "healthy," and we Americans fall for it, hook line and sinker.

> **WARNING:**
> A side effect of some of these food additives is that they can change our brain chemistry, causing us to become addicted and gain body fat.

Could it be true? It is. In fact, while researching *Belly Fat Free*, I traveled the country and interviewed dozens of food chemists who work for various fast food companies and major food manufacturers. What I discovered made me downright angry…and it should infuriate you as well.

"Off the record," over and over again one food chemist after another told me that their supervisors and upper management specifically instructed them to create foods that were as highly addictive as possible. A sprinkle of trans fat and caffeine here; some MSG and high fructose corn syrup there. Mix in some artificial colors and flavoring, extra salt and sugar, and *voila*! You have a deadly health time bomb, disguised as a harmless treat that you and your family can't get enough of.

Here's a specific example. Let's say you have a big food manufacturer that wants to create cupcakes. Typically, that food manufacturer will have a group of food chemists create two different versions of a cupcake, and the chemists are given these instructions:

54   Belly Fat Free

1. The cupcakes must have a long shelf life so they can remain on grocery store shelves for months (or years) without going bad.

2. They must be highly "desirable" so men, women, and especially children will eat them and not get full quickly.

The food chemists then go about creating the most highly enticing (read: addictive) "treat" that will outlive all of us. They'll add a cocktail of chemicals to achieve this: high fructose corn syrup, caffeine, trans fats, MSG, artificial colors, flavors, preservatives, and as many refined carbohydrates as they can stuff into the pseudo-food.

At the end of this project, the food manufacturer will have two versions of the cupcake to choose from. They will then conduct shelf-life tests, during which they put the cupcake through all sorts of "experiments" to quickly age the food to make sure the preservatives won't allow the "treat" to break down as nature intended.

Then they have taste tests with consumer groups, having them rate which cupcake is the most "appealing" based on various characteristics, such as taste, color, sweetness, texture, and smell. What the food manufacturer is really trying to do here is figure out which version of the cupcake will be the most addictive so that consumers will gobble them up like crazy. Not only will this process wreak havoc on your waistline, but it will add up to optimal profits for the manufacturer, which means big raises for the CEO and upper management. Priorities, right?

Cupcakes are just an example. And don't think that junk foods and fast foods are the only culprits. The same procedure occurs when these companies make macaroni and cheese, crackers, snack bars, syrup, jelly, frozen dinners, cereals, ketchup, some canned fruits and vegetables, lunchmeats, and many other foods you may consider healthy.

Make no mistake, these obesity additives are no laughing matter. Did you know that many of the chemicals all too commonly found in today's foods can be just as addictive as alcohol, cigarettes, and even various street drugs?

Well, it's true. In fact, a recent study by Princeton University scientist Bart Hoebel showed that refined sugar (the top obesity additive) can be one of the most addictive substances of them all, producing a pattern of increased intake, signs of withdrawal, craving, and relapse—all hallmarks of addiction. Hoebel has shown that rats eating large amounts of sugar when hungry (a phenomenon he describes as sugar binging) undergo chemical changes in the brain that are similar to those produced by cocaine, morphine, and nicotine.

Think about your own life. Are there foods or drinks that "call your name" in your weakest moments—like maybe at night in front of the TV? Are there certain "treats" you can hardly resist when they're in your presence? Are there "goodies" that you continue to eat even after you're full?

I'm willing to bet there are. Although this brand of chemical addiction may not be common knowledge to the average American, I assure you it's no secret to the money-hungry food and beverage manufacturers. I believe that many of these companies *intentionally* create thousands of highly addictive products and pseudo-foods, which line our grocery shelves, stuff our school vending machines, and are distributed at the drive-thru windows of greasy fast food joints from sea to shining sea.

How Obesity Additives Cause Belly Fat

With all of this in mind, here are three ways obesity additives work to make our bellies bulge:

1. Two of these obesity additives interfere with a hormone called leptin that tells the brain we are full while eating.

2. Other obesity additives add fat by changing how our bodies use the calories we eat. They do this by increasing a fat-storing hormone called insulin. When this happens, calories are converted to fat instead of being stored as "muscle energy." This leads to fat deposits in all of our trouble areas—like under the chin, the backs of the arms, the belly, and the lower body.

3. Still other obesity additives actually make us addicted to them and cause us to eat uncontrollably. They do this by altering brain chemicals called neurotransmitters—just like a highly addictive drug does.

This scenario seems awfully familiar to me. Remember when the tobacco industry was finally exposed for knowingly covering up the truth about the dangers of tobacco use in the 1970s, 1980s, and 1990s? These companies were adding as much of a highly addictive and disease-causing ingredient (nicotine) into their tobacco products as possible. They had "chemists" who developed ways to manipulate nicotine in order to make it more rapidly absorbed by the body and, therefore, more addictive. In fact, Hollywood created a movie about this true story called *The Insider* (1999) starring Russell Crowe and Al Pacino.

Once the tobacco industry's actions were exposed, it became obvious that good ol' Joe Camel knew damn well that his product would cause hundreds of thousands (if not millions) of good folks to get sick and die. There were class-action lawsuits galore and the tobacco giants tried to cover up the truth—as they had for decades before—but they ended up losing hundreds of millions of dollars despite their high-priced lawyers and paper shredders.

To be honest with you, I don't think most of today's major food manufacturers are any better than their tobacco industry predecessors. They are well aware that if they add dirt-cheap, highly addictive, disease-causing ingredients to their products in just the right amounts, Americans will gobble them up while manufacturers laugh all the way to the bank.

Unfortunately, there's a hefty price to pay for this "business strategy." Many customers fall victim to food manufacturers' ploys, eventually becoming overweight, dying, or developing serious life-threatening diseases that they then have to try and control with potentially harmful medications.

But this is just me saying that these obesity additives are bad, right? WRONG. Here is a photo from a recent TV interview I did, which shows a pile of studies conducted by some of the world's top scientists and medical doctors, backing up my claims that the following obe-

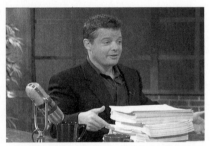

Here I am during a TV interview exposing the science on obesity additives.

sity additives are making us fat and sick…or worse. (A review of the science behind BFF is available at BellyFatFree.com/Science.) Let me introduce some of these studies, along with the seven obesity additives, to you now.

So how do you protect yourself? Outsmart the food manufacturers by educating yourself and staying away from these seven particularly dangerous—and all-too-common—obesity additives.

Obesity Additive #1: Stripped Carbohydrates: Sugar, Sugar Everywhere

It's crazy, really. Man takes sugar cane or vegetables like corn or beets (which are full of fiber and various vitamins and minerals in their natural state), and completely strips them of all health-promoting properties. What's left is a fast-digesting, highly addictive, nutritionally *dead* food that causes sickness and even premature death when consumed in excess. Of course I'm talking about sugar and, in the case of wheat, white flour. Contrary to popular belief, "stripped carbohydrates" as I call them (in all their various forms like sugar [sucrose], flour, enriched white flour, enriched bleached flour, enriched wheat flour, wheat flour, semolina flour, white rice, maltodextrin, glucose, fructose, malt syrup, corn starch, dextrose, and levulose) are really America's most fattening and dangerous obesity addictives. Although, ironically, most processed, "fat-free" foods are loaded to the gills with them.

Out of all the obesity additives, sugar is public enemy number one. On average, my calculations show that an average American eats **140 pounds of sugar per year—about 173 grams per day**. That's one tragic sugar addiction. It's important to know that sugar induces hunger and cravings because it wreaks havoc on your blood sugar levels, causing them to rise, then fall. When you eat

The Obesity Conspiracy Exposed   59 sugar, a surge of a fat-storing hormone called insulin is released into your digestive tract. Insulin grabs hold of this sugar and stores it as energy—and then that excess is stuffed into your fat cells in all of those dreaded trouble spots—like your belly. As a result, your blood sugar levels drop, causing more hunger and cravings. Then the vicious cycle repeats. (It's important to note that in the presence of insulin, the hormone responsible for burning body fat, glucagon, is "shut off." That's why chronic, high insulin levels will make it impossible for you to release belly fat.)

And if that's not enough to scare you off the stuff, recent studies have shown that sugar causes inflammation in your body that is the root of most disease. It also accelerates aging and wrinkles according to a study published in the *British Journal of Dermatology*.

And if you've noticed that you're feeling down lately, Annette Nay, Ph.D. says that sugar may be to blame in her 2007 article on sugar addiction and depression. Eating large doses of sugar during the day actually slows down your body's natural endorphin ("feel good" hormone) production, causing you to struggle with depression. To get out of the "sugar blues" we go straight back to the problem source, relying on more sugar to get us out of our slump. No wonder we can't get enough.

Here's something else to keep in mind: four grams of sugar equals one teaspoon of sugar. So when you look at a soft drink can (or any other energy drink or fruit juice) and see 40 grams of sugar in a 12-ounce container, this means you're drinking the equivalent of 10 teaspoons of sugar. That's right. There's no

> **Tip:** A bread is *not* whole wheat unless the packaging says "100% whole wheat." Otherwise, it is nutritionally the same as plain white bread.

difference between drinking a sugar-filled beverage and dumping 10 teaspoons of sugar into a glass of water and chugging it down. And where do you think all that excess sugar goes? If you said it converts to fat and is stored in your belly, thighs, hips, face, arms, and all those other trouble spots, you're right.

Now consider this. A 12-ounce soft drink (the same goes for energy drinks and fruit juices) has around 140 calories—all of which come from sugar—and the typical American has at least three of these drinks a day (yes, Starbucks drinks are loaded with fat and sugar too). Do you know how many pounds of blubbery fat this adds up to in a year if these calories exceed what you need in a day?

> There's no difference between drinking a sugar-filled beverage and dumping 10 teaspoons of sugar into a glass of water and chugging it down.

Roughly 44 pounds of fat.

It's no surprise that a recent study published in the *Journal of Clinical Investigation* concluded that ingesting fructose-sweetened soft drinks increases belly fat in overweight subjects. Other studies show a direct correlation between an increase in sugary soft drink consumption and type 2 diabetes and cardio-vascular risk factors.

Terrifying, isn't it? Are you starting to see why these sugar-filled drinks may not be a good choice? Are you starting to realize that maybe those extra pounds on your belly are not only because of what you've been eating…but also what you've been *drinking*? Are you starting to see why soft drinks, energy drinks, and fruit juices are not the best choice for children? Hmm…

And I'm not the only one talking about the dangers of sugar. The American Heart Association recently came out with a "warning" to Americans, published in *Circulation: Journal of the American Heart Association*. Lead author Rachel K. Johnson, Ph.D., M.P.H., R.D., professor of nutrition at the University of Vermont in Burlington, concluded that:

- ✔ High intake of added sugars is implicated in numerous poor health conditions, including obesity, high blood pressure, and other risk factors for heart disease and stroke.

- ✔ Added sugars and solid fats in food, as well as alcoholic beverages, are categorized as "discretionary calories" and should be eaten sparingly.

- ✔ Most American women should consume no more than 100 calories (25 grams) of added sugars per day; most men, no more than 150 calories (37.5 grams).

- ✔ Soft drinks and other sugar-sweetened beverages are the number-one source of added sugars in the American diet.

How much sugar is okay? With new research, like the study I just mentioned by the AHA as my reference point, and to make it simple, I recommend that men, women, and children who are interested in losing belly fat get no more than 30 grams of sugar a day (this includes natural sources from milk, fruits, and vegetables, too). This isn't a lot of sugar when you consider that the average soft drink contains a whopping 40 grams of the stuff. That's more than the amount of sugar that one should have in an entire day right there. (Now some of you may be saying, "30 grams of sugar is fine. I'll just use all of the artificial sweeteners out there instead." Think again. See the Obesity Additive #2 section for details.)

But I have to be honest. I'm not the type of person who is going to count sugar grams all day long. Let's face it, it's a hassle and it's not something most busy people can do for life. That's why I don't recommend that you count the grams of sugar you eat. Instead, stick to the BFF Recommended Foods I outline in Chapter 7 and you'll start losing that belly fat in no time…flat.

High Fructose Corn Syrup (HFCS)

Although high fructose corn syrup falls under the "stripped carbohydrate" obesity additive category, its huge impact on belly fat calls for its own "shout out." Now, HFCS may sound healthy (it *is* made from corn, after all), but it's not. This dirt cheap, man-made sweetener shuts down leptin, a fat-regulating hormone in your body that is responsible for sending "hunger signals" from your stomach to your brain. Essentially leptin lets you know when you're full. And when your brain doesn't get the message, you keep eating and eating and eating while the manufacturers of high fructose corn syrup, and the products that contain it, keep making more and more and more money.

Here's an example from a recent study. Test subjects were divided into two groups—one was given a glucose beverage to add to their diet, while the other group was given a beverage containing high fructose corn syrup to add to their diets. While both test groups gained weight, the group consuming high fructose corn syrup packed on intra-abdominal fat (or belly fat). And why is that so startling? It's because this particular kind of fat causes diabetes and heart disease. So, not only is high fructose corn syrup causing you to eat more than you should, it is literally putting your health at risk.

According to the U.S. Department of Agriculture, the average American consumes 42 pounds of HFCS a year. That's more than 75,000 empty calories that have *no* nutritional value! What's more, teenagers are consuming 15 to 20 teaspoons of HFCS a day when they need to be eating nutrient-dense foods for growth and life-long health. It's no wonder that *The American Journal of Clinical Nutrition* says that HFCS use increased by 4,000% between 1970 and 1990. The manufacturers of HFCS really are cashing in big... just like drug dealers...while America is adding belly fat at a very dangerous rate.

Speaking of a drug, have you ever indulged in a sweet dessert that just wouldn't fill you up no matter how much you ate? One of those treats that you have no self-control over, like, oh, I don't know...maybe soft drinks, fruit juices, energy drinks, ice cream, pudding, jellies, most "fat-free" foods, chocolate, crackers, cereals, syrups, candies, or desserts? If that's the case, you may want to check out the food label. Chances are it contains a large amount of high fructose corn syrup.

And remember, on American food labels ingredients are listed in order of the most abundant to the least (for more information on food labels, turn to page 91). So if, for example, you see HFCS listed anywhere in the first five ingredients, that's not good. You'll want to choose a version that doesn't contain HFCS at all or, at the very least, has it listed further down on the ingredients listing.

Obesity Additive #2: Artificial Sweeteners

Artificial sweeteners like Splenda (sucralose), NutraSweet (aspartame), Sunette (acesulfame K), and Sweet 'N Low (saccharin) may have serious health consequences and may be causing you to GAIN weight, not lose it.

One University of Texas-San Antonio study linked increased consumption of artificially sweetened diet soda with obesity. (Most diet sodas contain aspartame; a few contain sucralose or other sweeteners.) "On average, for each diet soft drink our participants drank per day, they were 65 percent more likely to become overweight during the next seven to eight years and 41 percent more likely to become obese," said Sharon Fowler, MPH, faculty associate in the division of clinical epidemiology.

Also, in a study published in the *International Journal of Obesity*, researchers fed one group of rats a liquid sweetened with real sugar, and then fed another group of rats a liquid mixed with artificial sweeteners. When they offered both groups food, the rats in the artificial sweetener group ate more.

Why? The scientists believe that artificial sweeteners may "short-circuit" the body's natural ability to sense how much it has eaten. They foil the efforts of our body's internal calorie counter, so we eat more without realizing it. It could also be that eating and drinking "diet foods" with artificial sweeteners makes us feel entitled to overeat at other times of the day.

Possible weight gain aside, these sweeteners may be harmful. The Center For Science in the Public Interest (CSPI) has aspartame, saccharin, and acesulfame K labeled "Avoid" in their guide to food additives, due to results of research that show a possible risk from these sweeteners. Aspartame (NutraSweet) in particular has been linked to tumors in several Italian studies.

Splenda (sucralose), which originally was marketed as being "made from sugar," actually contains chlorine atoms. Chlorine is used to kill microorganisms in water in swimming pools, and to a much lesser extent, in public water supplies. And in a recent Duke University study, rats who were fed food containing sucralose for 12 weeks had much less gut flora than normal rats. This means that the sucralose "killed off" the good bacteria that normally live in the intestines. These good bacteria, as we'll discuss later on,

> **Tip:** It's best to question any ingredient you don't recognize on a food label until you determine exactly what it is. To keep things even more simple, just put the food item in question back on the shelf and buy something else with ingredients you recognize and know are good for you.

have a *big* impact on your overall health and belly bulge. So you don't want to kill them.

Why take chances with your weight and your health? I recommend the new zero- or low-calorie sweeteners like truvia™, Z-Sweet®, and Sun Crystals™ that are made with natural sources, such as erythritol and stevia. You can find these at most grocery stores. These natural sweeteners can be used instead of sugar packets in your hot beverages, on oatmeal, and even in baked goods to some extent.

Erythritol is an all-natural, zero-calorie sweetener that is fermented from sugars and found naturally in many fruits and vegetables. It has no calories, no glycemic impact, and is only slightly sweeter than real sugar. It is recognized as safe by the FDA. Other sugar alcohols (such as xylitol or maltitol) frequently are blamed for side effects like gas and diarrhea when people overdo sugar-free treats. However, erythritol is absorbed before it reaches the large intestine, so it does not normally cause these digestive effects. In the U.S., the granular form is marketed under the name Z-Sweet® and found in other natural sweeteners including Sun Crystals™ (which is a mixture of erythritol and raw cane sugar so it's not zero-calorie) and truvia™ (which contains a mixture of erythritol and stevia).

Stevia rebaudiana is a leaf that first gained popularity in South America as a no-calorie, natural sweetener with a sweetness that is 30-45 times greater than that of table sugar. It's been used all over the world for years as a safe, natural no-calorie sweetener.

After a long debate (which many people believe was due to the chemical sweetener industry trying to block it), it's been approved for use in the United States. You can find stevia under the names PureVia™, SweetLeaf™, and mixed with erythritol in truvia™.

It's important to remember that you should use all sugar alternatives, even natural ones, sparingly. Let your body learn that it doesn't need sweets all the time to be satisfied, and you'll be on the fast track to better health.

Obesity Additive #3: Caffeine

To give caffeine a fair shake, various studies show that, in moderate amounts, it can assist with the breakdown of fat. However, most food manufacturers don't exercise such moderation, adding huge amounts of caffeine to their products to enslave you to their high-calorie foods and beverages that just add unwanted weight to your belly.

Case in point: A study appearing in the journal *Metabolism* concluded that (paraphrasing here)…excessive caffeine consumption can stimulate the adrenal glands into producing stress hormones, including cortisol, the hormone responsible for causing belly fat.

Other studies show that:

✔ Caffeine ingestion can increase stress that leads to overeating or binge eating.

✔ Elevation of stress hormones leads to fat cravings.

- ✔ Increased levels of the stress hormone cortisol increase appetite.

- ✔ Caffeine interferes with a "brain chemical" called GABA, preventing it from performing its calming actions. This can lead to "stress eating."

And a study published in the *American Journal of Clinical Nutrition* showed that caffeine use increases the insulin response to a sugar. (Higher insulin levels mean more belly fat.)

Make no mistake, caffeine is highly addictive too. In fact, if caffeine were introduced as a new food additive today, there is no way the FDA would approve its use because once in your body it acts more like a drug than a food additive.

Want proof? If you're a caffeine drinker (i.e., if you drink coffee, soft drinks, or energy drinks), go "cold turkey" tomorrow and see what happens. Within a few hours you may notice that your hands are shaking and you feel tired and lethargic. You may find it difficult to focus; you may even feel irritable and moody. And that's just after a few hours.

Now try going a few days without caffeine and you will likely get severe caffeine withdrawal headaches and begin to develop a lot of the same withdrawal symptoms someone coming off an illegal street drug like meth or cocaine might experience. Do you really think an ingredient that causes these side effects is healthy?

Roland Griffiths, a professor in the departments of psychiatry and neuroscience at the Johns Hopkins School of Medicine, is quoted in *U.S. News & World Report* as saying, "…the basic mechanisms by which caffeine hooks people is very much like our classic drugs of addiction."

Here's a quick story to illustrate my point. My dear Grandma Ruby used to drink a pot of coffee each and every day. In each mug she would add high-calorie ingredients like creamers and sugar. One day, my grandma was admitted to the hospital for some medical testing and after a few days she started to develop severe migraine headaches, shaky hands, irritability, and mood swings. The doctors couldn't figure out what in the world was wrong with her. Soon they started giving her a barrage of different drugs in an attempt to combat her symptoms. Well, it turns out she was simply going through caffeine withdrawal; after a few cups of coffee she was back to her normal, chipper self.

So let me ask you…why do you think coffee, soft drink, and energy drink manufacturers want to cram as much caffeine into each and every ounce of their beverages as possible? If you guessed it's because they're trying to addict you to their high-calorie product so you keep buying more and more, you hit the nail on the head.

Now don't get me wrong. A few cups of coffee or tea during the day are fine (certain teas, like green tea, actually have health-promoting benefits). However, when you start dumping obesity additives like sugars and fattening creams into these drinks it can really start to deteriorate your waistline, health, and overall energy levels.

According to MayoClinic.com, for most people, 200 to 300 milligrams of caffeine a day aren't harmful. A typical coffee will have 50 to 150 mg. Teas are 10 to 120 mg. Energy drinks are 80 to 150 mg. And most soft drinks have 20 to 50 mg of caffeine. But if you're experiencing any of these common side effects, you should continue reducing the amount of caffeine you're consuming:

✔ Weight gain
✔ Insomnia

- ✔ Nervousness/anxiety/restlessness
- ✔ Irritability
- ✔ Nausea or other gastrointestinal problems
- ✔ Fast or irregular heartbeat
- ✔ Muscle tremors
- ✔ Headaches

Obesity Additive #4: High Saturated Fat Foods

A few years ago, I saw CNN anchorman Anderson Cooper interviewing Dr. Marc Siegel of the New York University Medical Center. The good doctor was discussing all the new studies demonstrating that high-fat foods were as addicting as certain street drugs. In fact, he said, high-fat foods actually alter our brain chemistry, causing a surge in certain hormones that leave us wanting more and more fat. Dr. Siegel also brought up a study done at Rockefeller University that showed kids who ate high-fat foods craved more fat. This, of course, would lead to overweight children.

Make no mistake, I'm not talking about moderate amounts of good fats like you find in olive oil or flax oil, nuts, and avocados. I'm talking about the high amounts of saturated fats that are found in fast foods, dairy products (choose the low-fat versions), many processed foods, fatty meats, and typical junk food. Abuse of these saturated fats can clog your arteries, restrict blood flow, and can even cause heart attacks and strokes.

This is why the American Heart Association recommends that your daily saturated fat intake not exceed 16 percent of your total calorie intake. For the average 2,000-calorie diet, this is 16 grams (or less) of saturated fat per day. Store that in your back pocket, because there's no need to count fat grams with Belly Fat Free —I'll show you a better way to monitor your food intake in Chapter 7.

Hydrogenated Oils/Trans Fats

Trans fats are actually forms of saturated fats and fall under that obesity additive category, but just like HFCS, this obesity additive definitely needs to be called out on the carpet separately.

Do you remember those food chemists who added all sorts of nasty obesity additives to foods to make them addictive? Well, their "chemical tinkering" has also created dangerous, Frankenstein fats (more commonly known as trans fats). Food chemists got the bright idea to take a healthy vegetable oil, put it in a laboratory, and bomb it with hydrogen atoms. This process is called hydrogenation, and what results is a mutated oil that becomes solid at room temperature. This in turn allows the food manufacturers to put this frightful fat into processed foods to prevent them from going rancid as quickly. Sounds like a great invention, right? **Wrong.**

What they didn't realize at the time (or maybe they did and didn't care) is that once they chemically altered this once-natural and healthy fat, it became highly toxic to the human body. In a nutshell, these hydrogenated fats change your cell membranes by making them hard and brittle. Soon they become dysfunctional and your body attacks these cells, causing inflammation that can lead to diabetes, heart disease, weight gain, and certain cancers.

For example, a 2008 University of Paris-South study linked a high trans fat intake to a higher risk of breast cancer. Furthermore, a 2008 University of North Carolina study found that a higher intake of trans fats was associated with a higher incidence of precancerous growths in the colon.

Trans fats were also shown to increase LDL (bad cholesterol) and decrease HDL (good cholesterol) in a study published in *The Journal of Nutrition*. Furthermore, trans fats are directly linked to premature aging and obesity.

In 2006, a study conducted at Wake Forest University showed that trans fats actually redistributed body fat from other parts of the body to the belly. As I mentioned before, belly fat is the most dangerous kind of body fat because it's linked to heart disease, diabetes, and certain cancers.

Because of these findings, trans fats have been banned throughout much of Europe and, more recently, New York City banned restaurants from cooking with trans fats.

So why in the world are these bad fats still being widely used in millions of American restaurants and grocery store foods today? Why isn't our government doing more to protect us? The answer: High-priced food lobbyists in Washington are paid big bucks to protect the financial interests of their clients, the giant food manufacturers. Unfortunately, they are *not* protecting the health and welfare of the typical American citizen—even though we pay their salaries with our tax dollars. Even more unfortunate, Washington is basically ruled by lobbyists, special interest groups, and big business. We're just pawns in their game. But we can fight back by not buying foods with these obesity additives like trans fats/hydrogenated oils in them.

Obesity Additive #5: Monosodium Glutamate (MSG)

If you're like most people, when you think of monosodium glutamate (MSG) you think of Chinese food. But this innocent-sounding additive also lurks in a surprisingly lengthy laundry list of food products and ingredients.

MSG is a flavor enhancer, one of the most common food additives, and a staple in the Standard American Diet, which has a very fitting acronym (SAD). It shows up in all sorts of places, both obvious and hidden. For example, MSG is often disguised on food labels as "natural flavors"). MSG is one of the biggest enemies to those who are trying to attain (and maintain) an ideal weight. Numerous studies have linked MSG intake with unhealthy weight levels and obesity.

Animal studies show that MSG can cause lesions in the hypothalamus region of the brain and leptin resistance (meaning tested animals don't respond to the hormone signal letting them know they're full), which leads to unhealthy weight gain. Then there are other studies that show mice become overweight when injected with MSG.

Still more research demonstrates that in a study where calorie consumption and exercise were equal, the group of men and women who used MSG was more likely to be overweight than the group that did not.

Another study performed by the University of North Carolina showed a correlation between MSG intake and obesity in Chinese adults. They found that the study group who used the most MSG was three times more likely to be overweight than nonusers.

Need more proof that you should avoid MSG at all costs? In addition to being tied to obesity, MSG is likely associated with numerous other serious symptoms and health conditions including: diabetes, depression, heart disease, cancer, celiac, migraines, digestive upsets, infertility, ADD, inflammation, and possibly even asthma.

MSG may also be addictive. It affects a neurotransmitter (chemical messenger) called GABA, which stimulates the brain. A desire for this sensation can, in turn, cause MSG addiction. Convinced yet? Despite these studies and scientists' warnings to "…abstain from adding the popular flavoring agent MSG," this obesity additive keeps popping up in many processed foods.

Now that you're in the know, the next step is to avoid MSG; unfortunately, this isn't always easy. As we've already discussed, not only are tons of foods loaded with MSG in obvious ways (meaning a food label clearly states that MSG or monosodium glutamate is included), but MSG is also hidden in many foods.

To save you from the detective work necessary to hunt down these ingredients, here's a list of some culprits. (Keep in mind that some of the following items always contain MSG, while others may or may not contain it. To be on the safe side, you should consider eliminating these items from your diet altogether.) Suspect ingredients include: monosodium glutamate, MSG, glutamate, yeast extract, hydrolyzed protein, glutamic acid, autolyzed yeast, and maltodextrin. There are others, but this is a good start.

Processed foods are much more likely to contain MSG, so steer as clear of them as you can. Also, try to avoid non-organic produce, because MSG-containing products are sometimes used as sprays and fertilizers for those fruits and vegetables. If nothing else, be sure to wash all produce carefully.

Obesity Additive #6: Excess Alcohol

You may be surprised to see alcohol on my list of obesity additives because the wine industry would have you believe that everybody should drink one glass of red wine per day for better health. What's more, beer companies spend almost $2 billion every year in their quest to convince you of how "light" their products are. And hard alcohol distributors constantly try to tell you how uncool you are if you're not slugging down their fermented concoctions that taste like watered-down gasoline with a twist of barley and a splash of hops. (That's why these hard liquors are often mixed with high-sugar drinks...to make them palatable.)

I remember the first drink of alcohol I ever had. My father gave me a sip of his beer and I was shocked...people really think this tastes good? All of those attractive people in beer commercials really get their incredible bodies drinking something that tastes *this bad*?

When you think about it, the marketing of alcohol is quite ironic. To make alcohol, large vats are filled with yeast (a fungus) and a form of sugar (red grapes, beets, malted barley, and so on). The fungus then feeds on the sugar source and excretes the byproduct— ethanol and carbon dioxide. (Shot of fungus excretion, anyone?) Alcohol manufacturers then take this crude-tasting, highly addictive toxic concoction, slap a label on it, and begin telling American children that they're not cool if they don't drink their version of fungus urine. "Sure it tastes bad…but keep drinking and you'll develop an addiction to it." Or, "Hey, mix some sugar with it to make it even more addictive." Talk about pulling the wool over the sheep's eyes.

I want to take a minute to let the cat out of the bag here: There are much healthier and lower-calorie ways to get antioxidants than ingesting red wine…and there's nothing light about light beer. As far as I'm concerned, alcohol does much more damage than good (I know from experience, believe me). And, whether you're thinking about it or not, these calories can add up in a big way. After all, they don't call it a beer belly for nothing. Let's take a look at the numbers, shall we?

- ✔ One light beer = 100 calories
- ✔ One regular imported beer = 160 calories
- ✔ One 4-ounce glass of red wine = 90 calories
- ✔ One wine cooler = 200 calories
- ✔ One 8-ounce margarita = 450 calories
- ✔ One shot of hard alcohol = 100 calories

So let's say you enjoy just one light beer after work every day, then maybe a couple more on the weekends (and who really drinks just one?). That adds up to an extra 700 calories per week; 2,800 calories per month; and 33,600 calories per year. Considering that 3,500 excess calories equal one pound of fat, we're talking about adding almost 10 pounds per year, just from one can of "light" beer a day. (And we all know people who drink much more than this.)

This doesn't even take into account the greasy, fried items that all too often go hand in hand with alcohol. Would you eat those cheese sticks, potato skins, chips, pizza, and hot wings if you weren't drinking? Maybe not.

Here's another point to consider: About 5,000 children die each year due to injuries related to underage drinking. It's obvious that kids need positive role models when it comes to abstaining from alcohol, which is a well-known gateway drug. It's also well known that underage drinkers are more likely to smoke cigarettes and try other, more harmful drugs later on.

When you realize that 2.5 *million* people were killed or injured in alcohol-related car accidents in 2007, it becomes clear that we as a society have a big, fat drinking problem. The bottom line is this: Regardless of the brainwashing attempts of alcohol advertisers, alcohol is *not healthy*. It can lead to liver damage, heart disease, and cancer, not to mention all of the other diseases related to consuming excess calories. Now I certainly don't want to be the "fun police" here, but I suggest avoiding alcohol as best you can—or at least limiting it to two drinks per week—as a general rule. If you can't avoid this highly addictive substance, it's time to seek out professional help.

Obesity Additive #7: Excess Salt (Sodium)

Sodium is something that the body needs to function properly—it's important for water balance and nerve function, among many other physiological functions. However, you only need a small amount each day—about 500 mg is plenty. You would eat this amount snacking on a serving of most chips, crackers, canned food items (especially soups and canned veggies), pickles, various cheeses, pretzels, or salted nuts. (Not to mention that condiments like ketchup and salad dressings are packed with sodium.)

The bottom line: Most Americans are eating WAY too much sodium (4,000 to 6,500 mg daily), and it's not only hurting their health, it's expanding their waistlines. In fact, the American Medical Association (AMA) is pushing the FDA to withdraw its designation of salt being a "safe" food additive. (They want Americans to cut their intake by half.)

To me, this is really no surprise. After all, big food manufacturers know salt is a very addictive substance. All they need to do is stuff more of it into processed foods and people will eat more… while the food companies make more. Case in point: Clinical research has shown that salt shares characteristics with addictive substances (like morphine, cocaine, and heroin), by causing our bodies to release feel-good "brain chemicals" when we eat it. This is why salt addictions are quite common and some people who are told to reduce salt consumption have a difficult time doing so and often experience cravings and withdrawal symptoms.

In addition, a 2006 Finnish study published in *Progress in Cardiovascular Diseases* found a link between increased salt intake and obesity. They noticed that between the 1980s and mid-1990s, the salt intake in the U.S. increased by more than 50% as the population began eating more and more processed foods. Now keep in mind that when people eat more salt, they naturally have the desire to drink more fluids to maintain the water balance in their bodies.

Well, guess what? Between 1977 and 2001, U.S. caloric intake from sweetened beverages (like the "fruit" drinks, soft drinks, and energy drinks that are typically full of sugar and high fructose corn syrup) increased by a whopping 135%. Wow, it doesn't take a rocket scientist to see that as food companies make food that is saltier, people consume more of it, and then slug down more super-sized sugary drinks to wash it all down.

If that weren't bad enough, a diet that has too much sodium is a leading cause of high blood pressure, which can lead to heart disease and stroke—diseases that also go hand in hand with obesity. High blood pressure (a reading over 140/85) is caused when too much salt enters the blood, making the blood thick like a salty sludge. To thin the blood, your body will dump extra water into your blood vessels—causing the *pressure* to increase as the blood vessels expand. African Americans, Hispanics, and obese men and women tend to have a higher sensitivity to sodium and are more prone to high blood pressure as a result.

How much salt is okay? If you're choosing your foods from the Belly Fat Free Approved Food Choices (see Chapter 7), you really don't need to worry about this. However, if you want to get technical, anything below 2,300 mg of sodium a day is excellent. If you are already at risk of high blood pressure, then you should limit your salt to less than 1,500 mg a day.

By the way, I encourage you to use unrefined salts like Celtic Sea Salt or pure Himalayan Pink Salt, because they have all 84 minerals (regular table salt has only two), and they don't go through the unhealthy refining process like regular table salt does.

WARNING: Many fast food and quick-service restaurant meals will put you over this "daily allowance" really quickly. For example, a McDonald's double cheeseburger and small fries contain 1,310 mg of sodium. A mesquite chicken salad from Chili's (which might seem healthy, right?) has 2,710 mg of sodium, and that's more than a healthy adult should eat in an entire day.

You can limit your salt intake by:

✔ Eating fewer processed foods

✔ Opting for frozen or fresh veggies instead of canned

✔ Buying fresh meats instead of canned, cured, or smoked

✔ Choosing low-sodium versions of soups and snacks like (baked) chips, pretzels, and cheeses

✔ Asking for unsalted entrees at restaurants

✔ Choosing foods that don't list salt/sodium in the first five ingredients

✔ Replacing your salt shaker at home with a salt-free herbal blend, like a blend I found online from The University of Illinois Thrifty Living Newsletter.

Salt-Free Herbal Blend

5 teaspoons onion powder
2 ½ teaspoons sweet paprika
2 ½ teaspoons dry mustard
2 ½ teaspoons garlic powder
1 ½ teaspoons thyme
1 teaspoon black pepper
¼ teaspoon celery seed
1 teaspoon cayenne pepper (optional)

Combine ingredients and mix well. Spoon into a shaker. Makes ⅓ cup.

Are You an Obesity Additive Addict?

After many of my students learn about the obesity additives that are in our food and beverage supply, they start to wonder if these chemicals may be playing a role in their weight struggles. The answer is "maybe," depending on their food choices and eating habits. Honestly answer the following questions to find out if you have an obesity additive addiction.

1. When you're stressed out, anxious, or depressed, do you often reach for certain comfort foods to help elevate or mellow your mood?

2. When you consume certain foods or drinks, do you find it hard to stop even though you know you've had enough?

3. Do you still have severe cravings for a particular type of food or drink that contains one of the obesity additives I mentioned earlier in this chapter, even after eating a full meal?

4. Has your lack of eating (or drinking) control caused you to gain unattractive body fat in unwanted places like your belly, hips, thighs, face, and arms?

5. If you try to cut out junk food, do you find you can only do so for a short while and that it takes a tremendous amount of willpower?

6. Have your eating (or drinking) habits negatively affected your self-esteem or relationships with those you love most?

If you answered "yes" to three or more of these questions, chances are you're addicted to the obesity additives found in the foods or drinks you are consuming on a daily basis. But don't worry, I can help you overcome these addictions and reclaim your body and life. Fast.

Junk Food Rehab: Seven Steps to Recovery

Escaping the grasp of obesity additives isn't always easy. That's why it's time for you to visit Junk Food Rehab. I find that it takes seven days of rehabilitation for most folks to overcome the power of the obesity additives outlined in this chapter. Here are your seven steps to breaking free:

1. **Reduce the seven obesity additives from your food supply.** For highly addictive additives like caffeine and sugar, you *can* go cold turkey, but some find they need to reduce their intake by half each week to avoid severe withdrawal side effects.

2. **Replace obesity additives with healthy alternatives.** There's no doubt you will crave sugar, but rather than relapsing with a king-size candy bar or soft drink, satisfy your urge with an antioxidant-packed chocolate bar with a 70% cocoa content (80% is too bitter for me). Instead of sneaking a super-sized soft drink for that caffeine high, have some green tea, or naturally flavored warm teas (without sugar or artificial sweeteners), which may still contain caffeine but in much smaller amounts. Or enjoy a soft drink alternative like Zevia, which can be found at Whole Foods and other health food stores. For all my product choices, visit BellyFatFree.com/GoodBad.

3. **Get active.** I've discovered that the best "jackhammer" for blasting away food addiction is exercise. Exercise releases feel-good hormones throughout your body just like obesity additives do. But instead of *making* you fat, exercise *burns* fat. Soon enough you will become addicted to the feelings you get from exercise. If you haven't been active, be sure to start out slowly. (Check out Chapter 9 for my BFF Transformation Program.)

4. **Find a powerful reason to change.** Here's a cold hard fact: If you don't have a powerful reason for avoiding the magnetic pull of obesity additives, they will continue to rule your life forever. You need to have a reason to avoid them. And that reason has to be more desirable to you than anything else. Maybe you want to look breathtaking for an upcoming reunion, graduation, wedding, vacation, or holiday. Maybe you want to fit into those "skinny jeans" that have been collecting dust in the back of your closet. Or maybe you have a serious health issue you want to overcome. I don't know what the exact reason is…but you do. And when you harness the power of that reason, eating an entire chocolate cake won't be nearly as appealing. (Read more about this topic in Chapter 3.)

5. **Get sleep.** Exhaustion makes cowards of us all. There are countless stories of men and women who were experiencing great weight loss results until they ran themselves ragged and woke up 10 pounds heavier with a slew of empty pizza boxes surrounding them. Make rest a priority. I suggest at least eight hours a night and moments of planned relaxation throughout the day.

6. **Avoid hunger, stay satisfied.** If you make the mistake of waiting to eat until you're starving, you're much more likely to eat too much and make bad nutritional decisions. Avoid this by keeping an emergency snack with you at all times (such as a healthy nutrition bar, a handful of almonds, or a piece of fruit). Eating a mini-meal every three hours is one of the keys to the Belly Fat Free Eating Program. (Get the scoop on the importance of mini-meals in Chapter 7.)

7. **Find your bliss.** When you're tired, angry, lonely, depressed, or stressed, it's easy to reach for a bag of toxic potato chips to feed your emotions. When you start to feel negative emotions overtaking your body…breathe. Take a moment to do some yoga or stretches, clear your mind, reset, and smile. This too shall pass. Emotional management is key to avoiding junk food relapse.

BFF Assignment #3 ☐
Operation Kitchen Makeover

Your third assignment, should you choose to accept it (and as long as you're taking the time to read this book, you may as well get the most out of it), is to perform a BFF Kitchen Makeover. I'm talking about removing all of the toxic food and sludge that is destroying you and your family's health and happiness.

The first step is to get "buy in" from your family. I can already hear some of you saying, "There is no way my husband/wife/child is going to let me throw out their favorite foods. There will be a revolt in my house if I do that!" Well, maybe it's time for a revolt—a revolt against the monstrous food and beverage companies that have enslaved your family to their health-destroying chemicals.

In all seriousness, my best advice is to sit down and have a sincere talk with your spouse (or significant other) to explain what you're learning in *Belly Fat Free*. Let him read a few chapters. Have him visit our Web site at BellyFatFree.com to learn about our mission to fight fat and slim down America. Then ask this question:

The Obesity Conspiracy Exposed   83

"Don't you agree this would help us as a couple and as a family?"

Then, as a united front (if you have children), have this same talk with them. Begin teaching them what you're learning. Get them excited and involved in helping you choose better food and beverage alternatives. Focus on health, not weight loss. Do this as a family project. I can't think of anything more *valuable* to the long-term health and happiness of you and those you care about most.

The next step in this BFF Assignment is for you and your family to go into your kitchen and start tossing all of the food and beverages that contain obesity additives within the first five ingredients of their food labels. (Remember, ingredients are listed on the label in order from the most abundant to the least. The ultimate goal is to altogether stop eating these bad additives, but reducing your intake of them is a big step in the right direction.)

Also, don't forget to *have fun* while you're doing this. Let everyone pitch in to help make the family healthier. Donate the foods you've decided to discard to a local food bank. But whatever you do, *get it out of your house*. After all, out of sight, out of mind, right? (Incidentally, that's why watching constant junk food commercials on TV has been proven to make us fatter.)

Finally, visit your local grocery store to find versions of your favorite foods that don't contain the following:

Obesity Additives Reminder

1. **Stripped Carbohydrates** (listed as sugar, flour, enriched white flour, white flour, enriched bleached flour, enriched wheat flour, wheat flour, semolina flour, white rice, maltodextrin, glucose, high fructose corn syrup (HFCS), fructose, sucrose, dextrose, and levulose)

2. **Artificial Sweeteners** (listed as Splenda (sucralose), NutraSweet (aspartame), Sunette (acesulfame K), and Sweet 'N Low (saccharin)

3. **Added Caffeine** in soft drinks and energy drinks (a few cups of green tea or coffee each day are fine)

4. **High Saturated Fats** (also listed as partially hydrogenated oils and trans fats)

5. **MSG** (also labeled as monosodium glutamate)

6. **Excess Alcohol** (if you must, one to two drinks per week)

7. **Excess Salt/Sodium** in chips, crackers, canned food items, pickles, various cheeses, pretzels, condiments, and salted nuts.

Buy This, Not That

Now that you're in Junk Food Rehab, I'll let you in on some alternative choices that will allow you to indulge in some great-tasting foods that are low in obesity additives.

I've put together a very extensive free report full of "Belly-Bulging" brands of foods and "Belly-Reducing" brands of foods—the good, bad, and ugly choices. Unfortunately we don't have room in this book to include them all so visit BellyFatFree.com/ GoodBad for your free special report today.

The Great Organic Debate

Although organic is often more expensive, it's also healthier— you won't find "toxic chemicals" in most organic selections. I shop at Whole Foods, but keep in mind that most grocery stores, and even Wal-Mart food centers, now have many organic food options at affordable prices. Check out BellyFatFree.com/GoodBad for details.

What's more, to avoid the unwanted antibiotics and growth hormones found in animal products these days, I buy all of my meat and dairy products from organic sources. To avoid pesticides I buy all "exposed" fruits and vegetables organically, as well. I do, however, buy fruits and vegetables that are protected by an exterior barrier like a peel, rind, or husk from the local grocery store if they're more economical. (Examples of these include: melons, citrus fruits, corn in the husk, and bananas.)

A non-profit group called The Environmental Working Group releases an annual report of the fruits and vegetables that are most likely to contain pesticides. They dubbed this group the "dirty dozen" and collect their information from more than 87,000 government tests. The most recent report shows that peaches top the list for most pesticides. Others include: apples, bell peppers, celery, cherries, nectarines, strawberries, kale, lettuce, imported grapes, carrots, and pears. So be sure to buy these produce items organically.

On the other hand, the 15 fruits and vegetables that are least likely to contain pesticide residue include: onion, avocado, sweet corn, pineapple, mango, asparagus, sweet peas, kiwi, eggplant, papaya, watermelon, broccoli, tomato, sweet potato, and cabbage.

You can save money by purchasing these items at a regular grocery store, if need be.

If your local organic markets are too expensive for your budget, don't despair. As a general rule, make sure to avoid purchasing a lot of processed foods and take care to thoroughly wash your fruits and vegetables. The important thing is to surround yourself with high-quality foods to nourish (not addict) your transforming body.

Grapefruit Is Great Food

The grapefruit diet that was so popular several years ago is a fad diet that refuses to go away. Consisting of mainly grapefruit (plus a little protein), it is a definitively unbalanced plan. However, recent scientific evidence shows that a grapefruit a day may indeed keep the body fat away.

Full of fiber (12 grams per whole grapefruit) and low on the glycemic index (meaning it digests slowly), grapefruit packs a lot of antioxidant punch in a small package. A recent study from the Scripps Clinic in San Diego studied the effects of both grapefruit extract and fresh grapefruit on 100 obese volunteers. After eating just 1 ½ grapefruits daily for 12 weeks, the fresh grapefruit group lost an average of 3.5 pounds while the placebo group lost less than half a pound.

Note: Grapefruit has been shown to prevent the absorption of several types of medications, so if you take any regular medications and would like to start incorporating grapefruit into your diet, check with your pharmacist or doctor first.

> **Tip:** Natural fruits, vegetables, lean meats, grains, and low-fat dairy products are going to be your best bets to avoid obesity additives, decrease body fat, and increase health and energy. Most of these ingredients are found on the outside perimeter of your local grocery store. When you start dipping into the interior grocery store aisles, you'll begin to find man-made, pre-packaged foods that are chock full of fattening and addicting chemicals.

The BFF Grocery List

To help you with your grocery shopping, I've created the Belly Fat Free Grocery List. This list of healthy and slimming foods goes hand-in-hand with the BFF Eating Plan (which you'll learn more about in Chapter 7). Simply choose the foods you need to buy from this list and you're on your way.

Dairy
- ❑ Butter (regular or yogurt-based; no margarine—it contains trans fats)
- ❑ Cheese (1% or less)
- ❑ Cottage cheese (1% or less)
- ❑ Milk (skim or 1%; try unsweetened almond milk, as it's low in sugar)
- ❑ Sour cream (reduced or no-fat)
- ❑ Yogurt (1% or less; low-sugar)

Proteins
- ❑ Bass
- ❑ Beef (extra-lean ground; try to eat organic, grass fed)
- ❑ Bluefish
- ❑ Buffalo

- ❑ Chicken breasts (free range)
- ❑ Cod
- ❑ Crab
- ❑ Eggs or egg substitutes
- ❑ Elk
- ❑ Grouper
- ❑ Haddock
- ❑ Halibut
- ❑ Lamb loin
- ❑ Liver (beef, calf, or chicken)
- ❑ Lobster
- ❑ Mahi-mahi
- ❑ Orange roughy
- ❑ Perch
- ❑ Pork tenderloin
- ❑ Red snapper
- ❑ Roast (arm or chuck)
- ❑ Salmon
- ❑ Scallops

- ❑ Scrod
- ❑ Shrimp
- ❑ Sole
- ❑ Sirloin (ground)
- ❑ Soy burger patty
- ❑ Steak (club, flank, round, sirloin, tenderloin, or T-bone filet; all fat trimmed)
- ❑ Swordfish
- ❑ Tilapia
- ❑ Trout
- ❑ Tuna (water-packed)
- ❑ Turkey breasts (extra-lean ground)
- ❑ Veal
- ❑ Venison
- ❑ Whitefish
- ❑ Yellow Tail

Color Carbs (Fruits)

- ❑ Apples
- ❑ Apricot
- ❑ Berries
- ❑ Cantaloupe
- ❑ Cherries
- ❑ Clementine oranges
- ❑ Grapefruit
- ❑ Grapes
- ❑ Honeydew melon
- ❑ Kiwi
- ❑ Lemons
- ❑ Limes
- ❑ Mango
- ❑ Nectarines
- ❑ Oranges
- ❑ Papaya
- ❑ Peaches

- ❑ Pears
- ❑ Pineapple
- ❑ Plums
- ❑ Prunes
- ❑ Tangerines
- ❑ Watermelon

Color Carbs (Vegetables)

- ❑ Asparagus
- ❑ Artichokes
- ❑ Bean sprouts
- ❑ Bell peppers
- ❑ Beets
- ❑ Broccoli
- ❑ Brussels sprouts
- ❑ Cabbage
- ❑ Cauliflower
- ❑ Celery
- ❑ Chard
- ❑ Cucumbers
- ❑ Collard or mustard greens
- ❑ Eggplant
- ❑ Garlic
- ❑ Kale
- ❑ Lettuce, endive, mixed greens
- ❑ Mushrooms
- ❑ Okra
- ❑ Onions
- ❑ Peas
- ❑ Radishes
- ❑ Rhubarb
- ❑ Spinach
- ❑ Snow peas
- ❑ String beans
- ❑ Yellow squash
- ❑ Tomatoes
- ❑ Zucchini

Energy Carbs
- ❑ Bananas
- ❑ Beans, lentils, or peas
- ❑ Bread (100% whole grain)
- ❑ Corn
- ❑ Couscous (whole wheat)
- ❑ Crackers (whole wheat like ak-mak, Kavli, Ryvita®, or Wasa®)
- ❑ Cream of wheat (long-cooking—not instant)
- ❑ Flour (whole wheat)
- ❑ Oatmeal (whole oats)
- ❑ Pasta (whole grain)
- ❑ Potatoes (red or sweet)
- ❑ Quinoa
- ❑ Rice (brown or wild)
- ❑ Tortillas (whole wheat, corn, or spelt)
- ❑ Wheat germ

Good Fats
- ❑ Avocados
- ❑ Almonds (raw, dry roasted, or almond butter)
- ❑ Cooking spray (olive oil)
- ❑ Flaxseeds or flaxseed oil
- ❑ Udo's Oil or Barlean's Omega Swirl Oils
- ❑ Olive oil
- ❑ Peanut butter (natural)
- ❑ Pumpkin seeds
- ❑ Walnuts

Condiments and Spices
- ❑ Ketchup (HFCS-free)
- ❑ Cinnamon
- ❑ Herbs (fresh)
- ❑ Mustard
- ❑ Salad dressing (no MSG, no corn syrup)
- ❑ Salsa
- ❑ Spices
- ❑ Syrup (HFCS-free)
- ❑ Tabasco (or your favorite hot sauce)
- ❑ Turmeric
- ❑ Vinegars

Now you're in the know about the deadly obesity additives hidden in the foods and beverages you're eating and drinking. Hopefully your BFF Kitchen Makeover assignment is under way, ridding your home of all those dangerous obesity additives so you can free yourself from belly fat. If not, be sure to start cleaning out your refrigerator and cupboards before we move on to the next chapter. Remember, I will show you what common food products are bad and what brands to replace them with in the report at BellyFatFree.com/GoodBad.

Deceptive Food Labels

Want proof that the government doesn't always have our best interest in mind? Look no further than food label laws. Get this: The government controls how our foods are labeled, right? So how can a can of cooking spray, which is 100 percent fat, claim that it contains zero grams of fat per serving?

That's a darn good question, and the answer is that our government allows food manufacturers to adjust the serving size on their labels and then round down the number of fat grams. In this case, the cooking spray manufacturer says that a serving size is only one-third of a second; thus there is no fat per serving. This is totally misleading. After all, everyone knows that when you coat a pan with cooking spray it usually takes several seconds.

Pam® Cooking Spray

Nutrition Facts

Serving Size About 1/3 Second Spray (.27g)
Servings Per Container About 529

Amount Per Serving

Calories 0	Calories from Fat 0

	% Daily Value*
Total Fat 0g	0%
Saturated Fat 0g	0%
Trans Fat 0g	
Cholesterol 0mg	0%
Sodium 0mg	0%
Total Carbohydrate 0g	0%
Protein 0g	0%

Ingredients: Canola Oil, Lecithin from Soybeans, Water, Rosemary Extract, Propellant

The Obesity Conspiracy Exposed

What's more, many products' packaging would lead consumers to believe they are trans fat-free. Look a little closer, though, and you'll see partially hydrogenated oil on the ingredient list—which just happens to be public enemy number one when it comes to trans fats. So what's going on, anyway? Well, food label laws allow manufacturers to say that a food is free from trans fats (on a per-servings basis) if the amount of trans fats is 0.5 grams or less. This means all the food manufacturers have to do is reduce the serving size to a level where they can round down and make the trans fat-free claim. That's akin to saying a nibble of watermelon is free from water. It makes no sense.

Lays® "Sour Cream & Onion"

Nutrition Facts

Serving Size 1 oz. (28g/About 17 chips)
Servings Per Container About 11

Amount Per Serving

Calories 160	Calories from Fat 90

	% Daily Value*
Total Fat 10g	15%
Saturated Fat 1g	5%
Polyunsaturated Fat 4.5g	
Monounsaturated Fat 4.5g	
Trans Fat 0g	
Cholesterol 0mg	0%
Sodium 210mg	9%
Total Carbohydrate 15g	5%
Dietary Fiber 1g	4%
Sugars 1g	
Protein 2g	

Ingredients: Potatoes, Sunflower Oil, Sour Cream & Onion Seasoning (Nonfat Milk Solids, less than 2% of the Following: Maltodextrin, Onion Powder, Whey, Salt, Sour Cream [Cream, Nonfat Milk, Cultures], Dextrose, Monosodium Glutamate, Palm Oil, Parsley, **Partially Hydrogenated Soybean and Cottonseed Oil**, Lactose, Whey Protein Isolate, Buttermilk Solids, Citric Acid, Natural and Artificial Flavor, Lactic Acid), and Salt.

Belly Fat Free

Here's another example. Lean ground turkey, a great choice, right? After all, it's turkey and it says 15 percent fat (or 85 percent fat-free) right there on the packaging. Wrong again. First of all, that 15 percent fat refers to the turkey being 15 percent fat *by weight* (in grams), not by calories. Remember, a gram of fat equals nine calories. A gram of protein and carbohydrates equals only four. So although a gram of fat weighs the same as a gram of protein or carbohydrate, its calories are more than double.

Bad Choice:

Ground Turkey
85% Fat Free

Nutrition Facts

Serving Size 4 oz. (112g)
Servings Per Container Varied

Amount Per Serving

Calories 220	Calories from Fat 150

	% Daily Value*
Total Fat 17g	**25%**
Saturated Fat 4.0g	**32%**
Trans Fat .0g	**0%**
Cholesterol 85mg	**29%**
Sodium 85mg	**3%**
Total Carbohydrate 0g	**0%**
Protein 20g	

When you look at the food label, you will quickly see that four ounces of this ground turkey has 20 grams of protein and a whopping 17 grams of fat. That's about as much as a greasy fast food hamburger. Not to mention that many people will eat double the recommended serving size in one sitting. Upon further examination, you'll also see that each 4-ounce serving has 220 calories, 150 of which come from fat

(150 ÷ 220 = 0.68 or 68 percent). This means that this "lean" ground turkey is 68 percent fat. Yuck.

On the other hand, if you were to buy lean ground turkey that contains *only white breast meat*, you'd only be eating 0.5 grams of fat per 4-ounce serving, with only 4 percent of the total calories from fat (5 ÷ 120 = 0.04). This is a great choice.

Good Choice:

Turkey Breast
99% Fat Free

Nutrition Facts

Serving Size 4 oz. (112g)
Servings Per Container Varied

Amount Per Serving

Calories 120	Calories from Fat 5

	% Daily Value*
Total Fat 0.5g	1%
Saturated Fat 0g	0%
Trans Fat 0g	
Cholesterol 70mg	23%
Sodium 55mg	2%
Total Carbohydrate 0g	0%
Protein 28g	56%

So what does all this mean? Should you bring a calculator to the grocery store with you? Well, sure. Why not? After all, it *is* your body and health we're talking about here. If nothing else, look at the total calories listed on the label and compare that with the calories from fat listing. If a 100-calorie serving size has 50 calories from fat, you know it's 50 percent fat and you should make a better choice. *Don't let the food manufacturers get in the way of the body you deserve!*

BFF Success Story
Kyle: A New Lease on Life Personally and Professionally

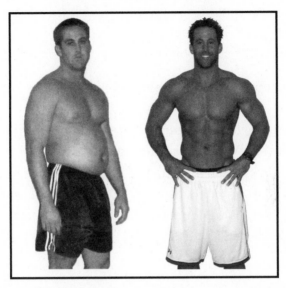

At age 35, Kyle Bonnstetter was your average desk-job junkie, slowly watching his youth (and his stomach muscles) disappear. Kyle hadn't been in good shape since college, and he wasn't living up to his potential. Not even close. Kyle says, "When I think about it, my lifestyle was destroying every area of my life."

Kyle had tried every workout. He'd bought every pill and tried every fad diet that came along for five years before successfully changing his body...and his life. Before he found Belly Fat Free, Kyle would manage to lose some weight every once in a while. But the minute he started eating "normally," he'd gain it all back...and then some. Then he'd get angry at himself and live on nothing but beer and pizza until he had no more pants to wear and was forced to do it all over again. Kyle always ended up tired, fat, and frustrated.

Finally, Kyle learned how to lose weight the right way with the Belly Fat Free Program. After just seven days, people at work noticed Kyle was losing weight. He noticed his abs starting to re-emerge, and after 28 days he had lost more weight than in the past five years combined! Changes trickled into other parts of Kyle's life as well, as he became more productive at work. These fast results really boosted his confidence and kept him motivated.

Ultimately Kyle lost 37 pounds in just 12 weeks. Now, he can finally walk into a room with his chin up. Kyle's results go way beyond just weight loss, though. He says, "People respect me and I respect myself. With my newfound confidence, I finally found success at work and in my personal life. I just took a VP position at my firm, I'm driving a new car, and just moved into a brand new house. Plus, I found my dream girl and married her. Life has never been sweeter!"

CHAPTER 5

Drug Deals and Slim Scams

Now we'll turn our attention to some of the other big money companies and institutions that work diligently day in and day out to ensure America gets and stays fat. We've already seen how food manufacturers contribute to the problem; now we'll take a look at how the big pharmaceuticals and weight loss scam companies do their part in propelling the obesity conspiracy.

Drug Deals

As we briefly touched upon at the beginning of Chapter 4, giant pharmaceutical companies don't make their money by curing what ails you. No, their profits come from ensuring you and thousands like you remain pill-popping clients for life. So when you go to a doctor with symptoms that may be weight-related, they don't give you a step-by-step plan for losing that weight. What they will do is start prescribing all sorts of different medications that many times are nothing more than dangerous Band-Aids designed to mask your real underlying problem—excess body fat caused by food addiction and lifestyle choices.

Check-in

Did you complete your third BFF Assignment (page 83), ridding your house of all the obesity additives that are destroying your shape, health, and energy levels?

If not, why not? As your BFF Coach I strongly encourage you to *take action right away*. After all, the health of you and your loved ones is hanging in the balance.

I hope you'll do that important assignment soon. (And by the way, if you're having some trouble with your family revolting against the idea of you tossing their favorite foods and exchanging them for different versions, take a moment to visit our forums at BellyFatFree.com to get support and advice from our members. We're all waiting to help.)

It doesn't stop with pills either. Recently doctors have been promoting procedures as well, some of which may be even more dangerous and unnecessary than the pills mentioned earlier in this chapter. "Restriction" surgery, for example, severely reduces the amount of food the patient can eat and also slows the speed with which food can leave the stomach. This surgery comes in a couple different versions. The first, commonly known as LAP-BAND®, can be surgically adjusted over time; vertical banded gastroplasty (also known as "stomach stapling") is permanent.

The most common weight reduction surgery in America today is the Roux-en-Y gastric bypass procedure. 140,000 desperate overweight patients turned to this surgery in 2005 alone. For this procedure, the surgeon opens the abdomen, creates a smaller stomach pouch with a stapler device, and connects it to the small intestine. The upper part of the small intestine is then reattached in a Y-shaped configuration. This surgery reduces the absorption of food and decreases the available size of the stomach.

According to the Mayo Clinic (MayoClinic.org), possible risks associated with weight-reduction surgery include:

- ✔ Pneumonia (risk increases post-operation)
- ✔ Blood clots in the leg
- ✔ Infections
- ✔ Hypoglycemia
- ✔ Leaks in the staple lines at the stomach
- ✔ Ulcers
- ✔ Hernia
- ✔ Anemia (due to deficiency of iron or vitamin B12)
- ✔ Neurological complications (from vitamin B12 deficiency)
- ✔ Kidney stone disease (due to changes in how the body absorbs calcium and oxalate)
- ✔ Possible bone disease (due to mineral or vitamin D deficiency)
- ✔ Dehydration
- ✔ Body aches
- ✔ Exhaustion or lack of energy
- ✔ Feeling cold in temperate conditions
- ✔ Dry skin
- ✔ Hair thinning and hair loss
- ✔ Changes in mood
- ✔ Relationship issues

Doesn't this seem a bit too risky and extreme to you? It sure does me. And that's why I'm on a crusade to get *Belly Fat Free* out to the doctors of America (more on this in a minute).

So here's a question for you: What happens to these hundreds of thousands of good folks who get gastric bypass but still can't control their appetites because of an underlying food addiction? Well, in some cases, patients literally burst their new stomachs, not surprisingly creating huge health risks. What's more, over time, many put the weight back on because they begin to stretch out their surgically reduced stomachs. After all, because these surgeries don't always involve education or the formulation of new, healthier habits, patients continue eating the same addictive foods they were consuming pre-surgery, which practically forces them to continue overeating.

Before finding BFF, many of my students considered going under the knife for these types of stomach-slaughtering surgeries (some even went so far as to have their surgeries scheduled). Luckily, they learned how they could naturally "shrink" their stomachs (learn how in Chapter 7) and how to overcome their addictions to obesity additives, ultimately losing the weight without surgery.

> Most doctors aren't required to take even one nutrition or exercise class during their entire medical education. That's completely insane.

Don't get me wrong—I don't mean to give doctors a bad rap. Most doctors are very concerned with the health of their patients and want to help them as much as possible. However, they're simply not trained in the area of weight loss. In fact, most doctors aren't required to take even one nutrition or exercise class during their entire medical education. That's completely insane.

Here's a quick story to illustrate my point. I have a friend named Dan who is a doctor. We went to college together and had many of the same science classes (although, in retrospect, Dan wasn't required to take any classes that focused on nutrition or exercise like I was). I recently ran into Dr. Dan at a class reunion, where we started discussing the obesity epidemic in America. Dr. Dan told me his biggest problem is the constraints that result from having only five to 10 minutes to spend with each of his patients. Obviously, this isn't enough time to teach anyone how to follow a proper eating and activity program.

What's more, Dr. Dan also said that he didn't feel comfortable teaching his patients about exercise and nutrition because he was overweight himself. Also, he hadn't taken any classes on nutrition throughout his entire medical schooling. (Note: A recent study showed that, like Dr. Dan, more than half of all doctors are overweight.)

Of course, I was completely floored by Dr. Dan's confession. He went on to explain that when an overweight patient comes in to see him, all he does is prescribe a medication or two to "cover up" the side effects. He also admitted this was *despite* the fact that he knew the real problem was the person's weight and the foods they were eating. Alternatively, Dr. Dan refers many obese patients to other doctors who specialize in gastric bypass surgeries.

When I informed Dr. Dan that effectively all he's doing is creating lifelong customers for the drug companies and (sometimes) promoting unnecessary surgeries, he agreed wholeheartedly and admitted that he was quite ashamed he wasn't doing all he could to help his patients. Dr. Dan was all ears when I explained the Belly Fat Free strategies I've taught my students. We exchanged contact information, and I followed up by sending him a few *Belly Fat Free* books to make available in his office waiting room.

A week later Dr. Dan called and said all of the books I'd sent him were already gone. He asked if he could get more copies so he could personally give them to his patients who wanted more information on how to lose weight the right way. Of course, I agreed and shipped him 50 more books.

Well, within a few weeks Dr. Dan called again, this time to report that many of his patients were losing impressive amounts of weight during the first week. He was amazed.

Dr. Dan went on to explain that he'd recently gone to a medical conference and, while presenting, he had shared his recent success stories with dozens of other doctors, calling for them to join him in standing up against the overmedication of America. He told me to expect calls from physicians around the nation who wanted to help their patients lose weight without medications or procedures, too.

> Soon, we started getting reports from various doctors whose patients had begun losing weight while following the healthy BFF lifestyle. What's more, some doctors reported that some of their patients were able to lower (or even completely stop using) a variety of different medications since losing their excess weight.

Sure enough, a few days later, my office started getting flooded with requests for *Belly Fat Free*. These good doctors were thrilled to have real, scientifically backed information to help their patients achieve their weight loss goals.

Soon, we started getting reports from various doctors whose patients had begun losing weight while following the healthy BFF lifestyle. What's more, some doctors reported that some of their patients were able to lower (or even completely stop using) a variety of different medications since losing their excess weight. (Note: Never stop taking a medication without your doctor's supervision.)

Doctors were even giving *Belly Fat Free* to the parents of over-weight and obese children so they could take action to increase their children's health and self-esteem. I can't tell you how proud I am of these parents for stepping up to make such a dramatic, positive impact on their children's lives. After all, studies show that 80 percent of overweight children become overweight adults. And the only way to stop this vicious cycle is through applied knowledge.

BFF Assignment #4 □
Operation Health Evaluation

This week I want you to call your doctor to schedule a complete health evaluation. Ask her to do blood work, and talk frankly to her about health issues that have been concerning you. Ladies, get a breast exam. Men, get your prostate checked. If you're 50 years or older or are in a high-risk category, get screened for colon cancer. I want to make sure you're in great health. And if you aren't, I want your doctor to catch it early so you have the best chance of getting healthy as quickly as possible.

Have your doctor review the medications you're taking and ask about the possibility of reducing or getting off these medications altogether (*always* with your doctor's supervision) as you begin to lose weight and elevate your health.

Join our free BFF online community at www.BellyFatFree.com

Keep the results from your health evaluation—I'd love to hear about your success. I know you will be amazed at the changes in your cholesterol, triglyceride levels, blood pressure, and pulse rates as you progress with the Belly Fat Free Program. When you follow BFF, I'm convinced you'll also see a dramatic transformation in your weight, energy levels, skin, hair, and even your mood.

And while you're visiting your doctor, be sure to talk to her about Belly Fat Free. Let her know you're following a safe and balanced program to lose weight the right way—by replacing bad foods with good foods and being more active.

By the way, help us spread the word by telling your doctor she can get a complimentary copy of *Belly Fat Free* by e-mailing us at Support@BellyFatFree.com.

Slim Scams

We've discussed the greasy food manufacturers and the drug giants, two of the industries that benefit most from keeping America obese. Now I want to talk about the weight loss scam artists who are preying on your hopes and dreams.

I'm sure you've seen it yourself. It seems every time you turn on your TV, open a magazine, or listen to the radio, there's a new "weight loss breakthrough" being touted. People get excited. Rumors spread that Hollywood celebs are using the latest and greatest product, whatever it may be. Magazines and TV shows start talking about this new fat-fighting breakthrough, using it to sell issues and get ratings. Soon, overweight Americans begin spending their hard-earned money to purchase the product in droves.

You too try this breakthrough product, but either nothing happens at all or you lose a few pounds, only to discover that the plan or product is impossible to use or to follow for life. (By the way, you should know that some diet plans and products even cause you to *gain weight* in the long run.) Rebound weight gain will only make you feel more disappointed and ashamed of your body than you were to start off with.

Weight Loss Scams Revealed

I'm sure you've experienced this scenario several times throughout your life. That's why I want to help you overcome these weight loss rip-off artists. I want to expose their sneaky tactics so you no longer fall victim to their overhyped promises and snake oil products. Following is a list of today's top five weight loss scams.

Scam #1:
Ab-zapping belts and gadgets.

Everyone wants a flat stomach and six-pack abs. That's why greedy advertisers constantly toy with our emotions, coming out with all sorts of abdominal gadgets, gizmos, and contraptions that allegedly transform our beer bellies into amazing works of art... and overnight to boot! If only it were that easy. But the reality is, it's just not. Despite this, millions of these products are sold every year.

Hands down, the strangest ab scam is the electronic belt that wraps around your stomach and electrifies your midsection. Allegedly this shock to your abs magically does away with belly fat, and almost instantly you're left with an amazing six pack. It's a miracle! Yeah, right. If refining abs is really this easy, why don't we all go stick our fingers in a light socket and become instantly slim? (Disclaimer: I'm not being serious, of course.)

When you see great-looking models wearing these ab belts on TV, keep in mind that this is probably the *first* time they've ever used the belt. Furthermore, know that the real way they developed an amazing midsection is by combining and timing their foods properly, avoiding high amounts of obesity additives, and moving their bodies intensely to burn stored body fat.

All those ab machines you see are really just a waste of your hard-earned money. The truth is, you can't spot reduce fat from your stomach by doing ab exercises with gadgets and gizmos. Think about it. Do you really think that you're going to be able to lie back in a "lounger" and rock your way to a set of spectacular abs in just a few minutes per day? Not a chance.

Ab loungers, rockers, swivels, gliders, beanbags…they're all a waste of time and money. I can't tell you how many homes I've been to that have these contraptions gathering dust in a closet or basement. (Maybe you have a few?) No matter what these advertisers say, instead of buying these crazy ab thingamajigs, you're much better off following the simple whole-body activity program explained in Chapter 9.

Scam #2:
Restrictive diet plans.

Here's a tip: If you can't follow an eating program for life, then you're setting yourself up for failure before you've even begun. Even if you do lose a few pounds initially, all the weight will come back and, most likely, you'll end up more overweight than you were when you started.

Cabbage soup diets, grapefruit diets, liquid diets, no-carb diets, no-fat diets, all-protein diets, soup diets, banana diets, black bean diets, Hollywood diets, marshmallow diets, they all have one thing in common—they don't work for long.

The reason? They're not a balanced, lifelong strategy. I can't tell you how many thousands upon thousands of letters, e-mails, and phone calls I've received over the years from desperate men and women who have tried the craziest diets you can imagine. It truly breaks my heart every time I hear one of these stories. After all, I've struggled with weight issues throughout my life and I've watched all my family members—my grandparents, father, mother, aunts, uncles, cousins, and two sisters—struggle with their weight as well.

I know what it's like to get ripped off. I know what it's like to feel desperate and hopeless. I know what it's like to spend money you don't have on the hope of a body you can finally take pride in. But please folks, I beg you, the next time you hear about a new breakthrough diet plan or product, keep just one thing in mind: **if it's not something you can do for life, you're not going to have long-term success.**

> **Tip:** Any successful eating program will include a wide array of fresh fruits and vegetables, grains, lean sources of protein (like low-fat meats or beans and nuts for vegetarians), and low-fat dairy products. If it doesn't, don't bother. You're just setting yourself up for heartache.

Scam #3:
"Too-good-to-be-true" weight loss miracles.

If a diet plan or product tells you you're going to experience "overnight results," turn around and run as fast as you can. I promise you it's a lie.

On a healthy weight loss program, most people lose an average of two to four pounds per week, depending on their weight, age, gender, and body chemistry. During the first few weeks, heavier individuals can lose seven or more pounds. (Note: Most people lose more weight in the first few weeks of any diet than they do in subsequent weeks.) What's more, if someone doesn't have a lot of weight to lose, they'll lose weight a little slower than someone who has a great deal to shed.

That's why some of the heavier contestants on TV shows like *The Biggest Loser* start off losing 10 to 15 pounds (or more) the first week. Sure, a lot of the weight they initially lose is water weight, but most of these men and women are also used to stuffing their bodies with thousands of excess calories each day. So when they get on a program where they're replacing bad foods with healthier alternatives and taking in the right amount of calories, they'll lose a great deal of weight quickly. (Not to mention they exercise nonstop on that TV show.)

In the category of "too-good-to-be-true" weight loss miracles, you typically see a lot of products such as liquid diet drinks, diet patches, and diet pills. Now I've got to be honest, some diet pills are truly backed by scientific research and they may help speed up a sluggish metabolism or provide the nutrients you may be lacking to help you burn fat faster.

But make no mistake, **there's no such thing as a magic bullet to instantly turn you "celebrity slim" overnight.** The real weight loss comes from changing what you eat (removing the obesity additives), when you eat, and your activity level. Period. (By the way, in Chapter 8 you can find my favorite picks for scientifically backed weight loss supplements that may help support and accelerate your weight loss efforts.)

And here's another tip: **diet patches plain don't work**—at least not the ones advertised by fly-by-night companies on the Internet and in some vitamin retail stores. You see, most of these diet patches don't contain any fat-fighting ingredients at all. And even if they did, there's no way your skin could absorb these ingredients—they're just too large, plain and simple. It's kind of like trying to eat lunch by lying down and placing a sandwich on your stomach; it's just not going to get to where it needs to go. Don't waste your money.

Scam #4:
Most pre-packaged diet foods and processed "fat-free" foods.

In theory, I like the idea of pre-packaged meals to assist in weight loss. They help keep portion sizes down, thus reducing the amount of calories eaten. But unfortunately that's about all I like about them.

You see, most of these pre-packaged foods (along with most processed "fat-free" foods) contain a wide array of obesity additives, such as high fructose corn syrup, refined sugars, MSG, and saturated fats. Plus, most of these foods are low in protein, which you need to stimulate your metabolism and build muscle tone. Not to mention the fact that they're packed to the gills with sodium, which can cause water retention and bloating.

In other words, most pre-packaged and diet foods I've seen out there are really low-quality "dead foods." Plus, they are extremely expensive.

Here's a question for you: What do you think happens when someone stops buying these pre-packaged foods? If she hasn't learned the proper way to combine foods and time her food intake, chances are she's going to return to her normal eating patterns and gain all that weight back.

So if you're thinking about using pre-packaged foods because of the convenience factor, just be sure to look at the ingredients and compare them to my list of obesity additives to make sure you're not consuming the wrong types of foods. After all, many pre-packaged diet foods are stuffed with obesity additives.

What's more, be sure to learn how to properly combine your foods and time your food intake (which we'll cover in Chapter 7) so you have the knowledge to lose weight and maintain that loss in the future, even when pre-packaged foods aren't available.

Scam #5:
Celebrity or fake doctor-endorsed diets.

Companies pay celebrities big money to promote products they oftentimes never even use. Here's a rule of thumb: If you wouldn't trust the celebrity in question to babysit your children, or balance your checkbook, don't trust her advice about a weight loss product. Especially when you *know* she's being paid to say what the company wants her to say. Just because an actress used to star in your favorite TV sitcom, doesn't mean she's qualified to give you weight loss advice. Remember, she has a whole behind-the-scenes team helping her get and stay slim.

Even worse than celebrities, some doctors are for hire. When you see an advertisement that features a doctor you've never heard of touting some new weight loss breakthrough, remember that he's being paid. And, just like some celebrities, there are doctors out there that will say anything for a buck or two. Besides, many of these "doctors" aren't the kind of medical professionals that the word conjures up. Many are doctors of dentistry, doctors of literature, or doctors in other fields that have little education in the areas of nutrition or weight loss.

So there you have it. The top five weight loss scams to avoid. Your next step is to find a powerful reason to transform your body. I wonder what yours will be?

BFF Assignment #5 ☐
Operation Scam Scrap

Here's a simple assignment. Go through your home and collect all the weight loss scams we've just covered that are hiding in your closets, shelves, pantry, garage, and under the beds. Now scrap them. That's right, throw them away. Whatever you do, just get them out of your home.

Believe me, there's something very therapeutic about doing this. You probably feel taken advantage of each time you see one of these scams in your personal space. Or you may feel like a failure because they didn't work for you.

It's time to move on and free yourself of these negative influences. It's time for a new beginning and real results. It's time for a new you. Sound good?

BFF Success Story
Tom: Father of Seven Slims Down and Discovers Inner Rock Star

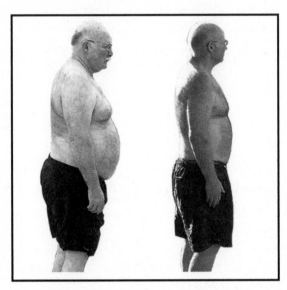

Before 55-year-old photographer Tom Potsko made a commitment to Belly Fat Free, he gave the entire program a thorough checkup and took it to his doctor for a second opinion. Not only did his doctor approve the program, he loved it. "This is exactly the way weight loss should be done," Tom's physician told him.

Tom also looked into a calorie-counting weight loss program, but he wondered, "Why do all the work of counting and adding up calories when the Belly Fat Free Cup Method™ (see Chapter 7) is so much easier and accomplishes the same thing?"

So Tom dove in, following the BFF Eating Plan™. However, the exercise program presented a challenge. In 1996, Tom had hip replacement surgery and he had also suffered from rheumatoid arthritis for more than 20 years. In the past, the pain inhibited his exercise plans and, in fact, had put the kibosh on his previous weight loss attempts. But with the support of the BellyFatFree.com community and the chance to win cash and a Caribbean cruise on the line in the BFF Challenge, Tom worked his way through every single difficulty that arose along the way.

"After the first six weeks, I lost 44 pounds and I decided I wanted to add upper-body exercises," he explains. "But having a left wrist nearly fused by arthritis and tendonitis, my options were limited. I chose lightweight barbells and some static exercises and hoped for the best. By week eight, the tendonitis pain started to fade, and I've had no pain since week nine. Now I've joined a gym so I can continue my muscle toning."

Tom decided to skip the optional weekly splurge meals (see Chapter 7). He said pasta is a big trigger for him, and it was easier if he didn't eat it at all. Twice during the 12 weeks, Tom's wife made her special spaghetti and he overate. "I had to work out extra hard after those meals. I adore her chili, too. So for me, it was best to avoid those foods."

Tom's persistence paid off. After just 12 weeks **he dropped 65 pounds of fat, trimmed 21½ inches from his body, and is down eight pant sizes.** His cholesterol went down from 238 to 172, and his triglycerides dropped from 111 to 64. Those are the numbers. But the real story is how Tom's life changed right along with his weight.

With his newfound energy, Tom no longer nods off during the afternoon. At night, he quickly falls into a peaceful sleep. No longer embarrassed about his weight, he is looking forward to a summer family reunion and a wedding. He walks the hills by his home with his grandchildren, no longer slowed down by an oversized belly.

And speaking of getting out and pursuing new interests, Tom hooked up with some friends and he now sings in a rock and roll band. How cool is that?

Belly Fat Free

CHAPTER 6

The BFF Commandments

Wouldn't it be fantastic if you could count on the constant barrage of information and advertisements about weight loss to be 100 percent true? It's a shame, but unfortunately it doesn't work that way.

Throughout the years, I've discovered that many people are extremely confused, frustrated, and downright misinformed when it comes to losing fat and shaping up—and who can blame them? After all, almost **everyone is feeding us false information.** And that's unsettling…not to mention detrimental to our collective health and belly bulge.

Weight Loss Lore

From the money-hungry advertisers who (as discussed in Chapter 5) are constantly peddling all sorts of "breakthrough" weight loss gimmicks and gadgets to celebrities pushing ridiculous diets (that they don't follow) to the deep-seated myths that have been passed from one generation to the next, we're constantly bombarded with inaccurate information. Some of which makes us even fatter and unhealthier.

Even most medical doctors don't have a clue about how to really lose weight and keep it off for life. They'll say something like, "You gotta eat right and exercise." But what does that really mean?

Then there's the giant food manufacturers discussed in Chapter 4; these companies are adding all sorts of addictive, hunger-inducing chemicals to food to keep your waistline and, more importantly, their profits growing.

It's no wonder that nine out of every 10 people who try to lose weight fail. (And that, my friend, is why I'm working so hard to give you the real scoop.) Have you failed to lose weight in the past? If so, it's quite possible that the failure wasn't really yours (although, trust me, I know it feels that way) but rather the program you were using. Believe me, no one can succeed while following bad advice. It's like trying to reach a specific destination with bad directions.

The BFF Commandments

So right here, right now, let's set the record straight. Let's clear our minds of all the mumbo-jumbo and misconceptions that have been force-fed to Americans over the years and replace them with information that will empower you to attain that new Belly Fat Free. The basics are included in the Belly Fat Free Commandments.

Commandment #1:
Reduce sugar intake.

Out of all the obesity additives, sugar is public enemy number one. On average, my calculations show that the typical American eats **140 pounds of sugar per year—about 173 grams per day**. That's one giant bag of sugar. It's important to know that sugar induces hunger and cravings because it wreaks havoc on your blood sugar levels, causing them to rise, then fall. When you eat sugar, a surge of a fat-storing hormone called insulin is released into your digestive tract. Insulin grabs hold of this sugar and stores it as energy—and then the excess is stuffed into your fat cells in all of those dreaded trouble spots—like your belly. As a result, your blood sugar levels drop, causing more hunger and cravings. Then the vicious cycle repeats.

And if that's not enough to scare you off the stuff, recent studies have shown that sugar creates inflammation in your body that is the cause of most disease. It lowers your immune system. It also accelerates aging and wrinkles. Not to mention that studies now say that sugar is as addictive as nicotine and cocaine. No wonder we can't get enough.

This is why, based on current research, I recommend that my students limit their sugar intake to a max of 30 grams a day (including natural sugars found in dairy products, fruits, and vegetables). But don't worry, I'm not recommending that you count sugar grams all day. Instead, stick to the BFF Recommended Foods I outline in Chapter 7 and you will naturally start consuming low amounts of sugar without the hassle. By the way, if you want to see a listing of my recommended low-sugar foods visit BellyFatFree.com/SugarFiber.

Commandment #2:
Eat more fiber.

Did you know that fiber (along with fats and proteins) fights belly fat by slowing down the absorption of sugar in the body and it helps to cleanse the belly bulge (waste) that comes from an overloaded digestive system?

Fifty percent of Americans aren't getting enough fiber from their daily diet. After all, the American Heart Association recommends 25 to 30 grams of fiber per day to reduce the risk of heart disease. However, most folks are getting only half of that, which is causing digestive problems and increasing their risk of heart disease, diabetes, and certain cancers.

Why is fiber so important for weight loss? Fiber-rich foods make you feel fuller for longer, and they slow the digestion of food so insulin (a fat-storing hormone) is released into the digestive tract. Plus, eating enough fiber (combined with eight to 10 glasses of water a day) keeps your digestive system running smoothly and can clean out pounds of "internal waste" that makes your belly bulge. Forget all of those unhealthy laxatives and cleansing detox pills you see advertised…all you really need is an adequate amount of fiber, water, and probiotics.

> Fifty percent of Americans aren't getting enough fiber from their daily diet.

My top choices for fiber-rich foods (more at BellyFatFree.com/SugarFiber):

- ✔ Barley has 12 grams per ½ cup
- ✔ Beans like black beans, navy beans, refried, and lima beans all have 6 or more grams per ½ cup
- ✔ Bran cereal has 13 grams per ⅓ to ½ cup
- ✔ Peas have more than 9 grams per ½ cup
- ✔ Corn on the cob has 5 grams per ear
- ✔ Strawberries have 4 grams per cup and raspberries have more than 5, and blackberries have more than 7 grams
- ✔ Potatoes with the skin—a medium-sized spud has 5 grams
- ✔ Broccoli has 7 grams per ¾ cooked cup
- ✔ Oatmeal has 7 grams per ¾ cup
- ✔ Apples have 4 grams of fiber in the form of pectin
- ✔ Dried fruits like figs and pears have more than 10 grams per ½ cup

Commandment #3:
Replenish your good bacteria.

Your body is supposed to be home to trillions of tiny bacteria. And that's a good thing. These beneficial microorganisms serve important functions within the body, mainly within the digestive tract. They do things like ferment foods that we cannot digest (such as fiber), help with elimination, support the immune system, prevent growth of harmful bacteria, and help the body absorb vitamins and minerals. What becomes a problem is when the toxins we have been consuming, as well as medicines like oral antibiotics, have a detrimental effect on these natural bacteria, also called "flora."

Obviously, when the intestinal environment is compromised, digestive side effects may occur. That's why it is common for people taking antibiotics to experience diarrhea, which a 2004 study from Pierre et Marie Curie University in Paris linked directly to the change in gut flora. When "good bacteria" are killed, "bad bacteria" are more likely to take their place and cause problems. A study I talked about in the section on artificial sweeteners found that eating food with Splenda for three months reduced the gut flora in rats. (Maybe it does this in humans, too?)

I recommend adding probiotics and prebiotics to your diet each day in order to maintain the best intestinal environment and reduce your belly bulge quickly. "Probiotics" are foods that either naturally, or because they have been added, contain quantities of beneficial bacteria. "Prebiotics" are foods that contain fiber, which provide nourishment for all those little bacteria.

I recommend sticking to sources that are as natural as possible. Here are some good probiotic foods to consider, and remember, most brands of yogurt contain excess sugar, HFCS, or artificial sweeteners. Avoid them!

✔ Stonyfield Farms Oikos Greek Yogurt (plain). Add a zero or low-calorie natural sweetener like truvia™ or Z-Sweet®. Add a high-fiber fruit like raspberries as a bonus.

✔ Lifeway Organic Kefir (plain). This is a drinkable yogurt. Add a splash of vanilla and cinnamon from your spice rack, plus a handful of your favorite high-fiber berries and natural sweetener, if desired. Blend. This makes a great smoothie!

As an alternative, consider trying one of the new shelf-stable probiotic pills, such as Align (Aligngi.com), or Culturelle (Culturelle.com).

Commandment #4:
Eat tasty foods every three hours.

A common mistake dieters make is assuming they will lose fat if they eat less frequently. Have you ever thought, "Hmmm… maybe I'll have just a small meal or two each day?" This seems like a logical plan, right? *Wrong.*

Believe me, it's the absolute worst approach. When you starve your body, it begins to fight back by conserving fat and burning muscle tissue. This dramatically slows your metabolic rate, which in turn *prevents fat loss.* Losing muscle tissue also leads to a loss of muscle tone and shape. Oh, and I should also mention that this approach ultimately makes you look flabby, not firm.

What's more, after a while a starvation diet makes you irritable, less focused, tired, and weak. Your health is compromised and your immune system is impaired, thanks to an inadequate supply of health-promoting nutrients. After a few days, fierce food cravings take over, binging follows, and you end up gaining back all of the weight you've lost…and more.

But even *that's* not the end of it. The next time you start dieting, the vicious cycle starts all over again. Only now your metabolism is even slower because, during the previous dieting episode, calorie-burning muscle was burned for energy. (By the way, each pound of muscle you lose while dieting causes you to burn about 50 calories *less* per day.) So now you have to eat even fewer calories than before to lose weight. (Ugh!)

This is what we call yo-yo dieting and it can wreak havoc on your body. A better alternative to starving yourself or skipping meals is to feed your body healthy foods every three hours throughout the day. By doing this your metabolism keeps burning calories at an accelerated pace all day long. Part of the reason this occurs is due to something called the *thermic effect of foods*.

> Feed your body healthy foods every three hours throughout the day to boost your metabolism naturally.

It works like this: Nutrient-dense foods tend to be more complex. Take proteins, for instance (lean meats, low-fat cottage cheese, and eggs). It takes more energy for your body to digest and use proteins than it does for simpler foods like sugars. The thermic effect of protein is the highest of all foods. After eating protein, your metabolic rate will increase by approximately 17 to 20 percent. In other words, if you eat 100 calories of protein, 17 to 20 of those will be burned just digesting and using the protein. By comparison, the thermic effect of carbohydrates is typically around 10 percent, and fat is just 5 percent.

Plus, by eating complex food more frequently (five mini-meals spaced three hours apart), your body will better use the nutrients you consume because they are in smaller quantities that are easy to break down and absorb. Too many calories ingested at once tends to overload your digestive system, so many valuable vitamins and minerals "escape" while extra macronutrients (carbs, proteins, and fats) are more likely to convert to body fat. Frequent healthy eating also helps stabilize blood sugar levels, which zaps excess hunger and cravings; limits fat storage (by limiting the actions of a fat-storing hormone called insulin); and reduces the energy drain that accompanies big meals.

Here's what I hope you'll take away from all of this: Eating five small, tasty, obesity-additive-free meals every three hours throughout the day is the quickest, most painless way to get slim for life. **It's my number-one nutrition tip for losing weight without depriving yourself of great-tasting food.**

By the way, if you don't already have *The Belly Fat Free Cookbook,* which is chock-full of more than 100 tasty BFF Recipes (already balanced correctly for you), you can get a copy by visiting us online at BellyFatFree.com/Cookbook.

Commandment #5:
Balanced meals are the key to your success.

If you're considering going on one of those low- or no-carbohydrate diets, please pay special attention to this next part. Following are just a few of the reasons why I **do not recommend** these crazy diets:

1. You can't follow this type of diet for life. Sooner or later you will fail because your body will fight you every step of the way.

2. Low-carb diets decrease a thyroid hormone (T3) that helps regulate your metabolism. So when you start eating carbohydrates again (and you *will*), you will likely gain back all of the belly fat you've lost...fast.

3. The quick weight loss you may experience on a no- (or low-) carb diet is usually attributed to a loss of body water and not body fat, which is, of course, only temporary.

4. You will begin breaking down muscle tissue for energy, which decreases muscle tone and further decreases your metabolism.

5. Cutting out fruits, vegetables, and grains (carbohydrates) robs your body of ample amounts of vitamins, minerals, fiber, and other nutrients that enhance and promote health. (And most of us don't get enough of these nutrients in the first place.)

As you can see, the low- or no-carb diet has many flaws that negatively impact your ability to succeed in getting that traffic-stopping body and keeping it for the long run.

Conversely, super high-carb diets aren't the solution either. High-carb diets tend to stimulate an excess amount of insulin production. Plus, high-carb diets are notoriously low in protein, which can have terrible consequences on your ability to build your muscles and shape your body.

And, if you're following some "point system" that allows you to eat whatever you want as long as you don't exceed your points, believe me, you are not getting the nutrients your body needs to be healthy and attractive.

The solution? I've discovered that a diet containing moderate amounts of protein (around 30 percent), moderate carbs (around 50 percent), and lower to moderate amounts of fat (around 20 percent) works best for most people and can easily be followed for life. But don't worry about these percentages. There's an easier way to keep track of what you're eating. I'll cover that next.

Commandment #6:
Count cups, not calories.

Have you ever been on a diet that required you to count every calorie or fat, carb, or protein gram you ate? I have. And, it works *only if* you have a solid grasp on nutrition and have the time and discipline to weigh and keep track of your food selections all day long. All of this takes a lot of work and can be very confusing.

That's why I recommend counting cups instead of calories. What are cups? I'm talking about measuring cups. And it works like a charm. Many weight loss gurus recommend counting portions, not calories. They say a portion of carbohydrates is an amount equal to the size of your clenched fist, while a serving of protein would fit in the palm of your hand with a thickness equal to that of a deck of playing cards. So a portion is going to vary in size depending on the size of your hand, right? Well, that's too general for this book.

I discovered that this "portion program" didn't work for a lot of people. They would eyeball a food item and somehow make every portion size they saw fit into the unspecific guidelines given. "That gigantic bagel looks to be the size of my fist." Or, "That turkey leg is about the size of my palm."

To avoid all of this, I designed my BFF Eating Plan around something very simple and specific—measuring cups. That way, there's no denying exactly what one cup of food is. My plan also takes body weight into consideration, which is crucial because the amount of food you eat at each meal is dependent upon that.

An even simpler way to achieve a nutritious, delicious, and balanced meal is by using a nutrition shake designed specifically for busy men and women. We'll talk more about all of this—including my new Belly Fat Free Cup Method™—in the BFF Eating Plan in Chapter 7.

Commandment #7:
Move your body.

The honest truth is that you can lose weight without doing any exercise. It's simply a matter of eating a few hundred calories less than you burn each day. However, this process takes *forever* and it does nothing in terms of firming or building up your body. Plus, by dieting without activity, as much as 50 percent of the weight you lose will come from muscle tissue—leaving you smaller but with less tone and a slower metabolism. (Not good.)

Adding some activity to your game plan can dramatically speed up your weight loss efforts. In fact, with activity, you can easily lose 200 to 300 percent more body fat while maintaining or increasing your muscle tone at the same time. (Bottom line: If you wanna transform your body, you gotta move your body.)

The key to success lies in finding an activity you truly enjoy; something that sparks your interest. And don't be afraid to cross-train (just a fancy word for trying something new if you get bored). The important thing is to vary your intensity levels while exercising. We'll cover all of this in full detail in Chapter 9.

If I had to choose the one exercise that gives you the most bang for your buck, it would be resistance training (lifting weights), hands down. Why? Well, for one thing, resistance training increases muscle tone, which in turn increases your metabolism (the rate at which your body burns calories) not only during exercise but 24 hours a day, every day. For example, Tina White, a former BFF Challenge Winner, gained six pounds of muscle during her transformation. This added muscle means Tina's body will automatically burn an extra 300 calories each and every day. Translation: Tina gets to eat more without gaining weight. Not a bad deal, I'm sure you'll agree. (To read more about Tina's transformation, turn to page xi.)

Secondly, resistance training actually changes your *shape*. It helps tighten and tone your body, including all those trouble areas. With resistance training, you can even change your proportions to make your waist or hips appear smaller compared to your shoulders. This is great news for those who currently have a pear shape.

> With resistance training, you can even change your proportions to make your waist or hips appear smaller compared to your shoulders.

Sometimes women are afraid they'll get big and bulky like a man if they train with weights. But, actually, the exact opposite is true. The Belly Fat Free Resistance Routine™ helps women achieve firm and feminine shapes and curves. For men, it helps build a strong, athletic, and Belly Fat Free body.

One last thing. You don't need to spend hour upon hour exercising. Nope. **Just 30 focused minutes a day is all it takes (and if you're new to exercise, I'm only asking for five minutes three times a week to start).** Not only that, but you can break up this time into smaller amounts (like three 10-minute sessions, for example), if that works better for you. I'll describe an exact program for you to follow in Chapter 9.

Commandment #8:
Lock up your scale.

Too many of us obsess when we get on the scale and see we've gained a few pounds. And when you're trying to lose weight, there's no faster way to ruin your day than to see the scales tipping in the wrong direction. Been there, done that.

When all is said and done and you've reached your goals, the scales will most likely register a loss—maybe even a big one. **But don't be surprised if your weight fluctuates a bit throughout the program.** In fact, I'd be surprised if it didn't. The time of day, your hydration level, the amount of waste in your digestive tract, and (if you're a woman) your monthly cycle will all affect the scale.

Moreover, one square inch of muscle tissue weighs more than the same amount of fat. So as you start toning your body and exchanging not-so-appealing fat for attractive muscle tone, the scale won't paint a true picture of the progress you're making at all. But the mirror will…and so will your loose-fitting clothes. A pound of fat takes up three times the space a pound of muscle does. So when you lose fat and add muscle you will drop inches.

Don't get me wrong. While I don't endorse the scale, I *do* think it's important to keep track of your weight loss progress. So here are some alternatives to using a scale every day:

1. Lock your scale away after recording your starting weight for the BFF Challenge. If you just *have* to weigh yourself, **don't do it more than once every week.** And remember, your weight can fluctuate as much as three to five pounds depending upon your hydration levels, the "trapped" waste in your belly, and the time of day. When you do weigh, do

it in the morning before eating or drinking, while wearing minimal clothing.

2. Take some "before" photos too so you can evaluate your progress each week. Yeah, I know these can be sort of intimidating, but it's vitally important for you to see what you *really* look like before starting the Challenge. (Most people don't realize how out of shape they are until they see themselves in a photo or video.) Believe me, these photos will be a real eye-opener and will give you the motivation necessary to stay on your program. Besides, you need those photos to participate in the BFF Challenge and get all those great prizes!

3. Take "before" tape measurements of all the important spots—your chest, waist, hips, thighs, and upper arms. Then you can re-measure these areas every few weeks. At the end of the program, you'll have a clear idea of how far you've come. (Fill out the Body Measurement Report Form in the BFF Challenge Rules and Regulations Guide at BellyFatFree.com/Challenge.)

Commandment #9:
Only use scientifically backed weight loss supplements.

It would be nice if there were miracle body-slimming pills or potions that would instantly transform us all into stunning supermodels or lean athletes overnight. Unfortunately, although many of today's dietary supplements would have you believe they can do exactly this, it's just not possible. Worst of all, many of these "miracle" potions don't even contain what the label may lead you to believe they do.

But there are certain scientifically backed products that may accelerate your progress when combined with exercise and a sensible eating plan. These supplements *may* boost metabolism, increase muscle tone, improve health, and help you shed unwanted inches at a surprising rate. I encourage you to learn more about these in Chapter 8.

Your body requires dozens upon dozens of nutrients—vitamins, minerals, trace elements, essential amino acids, and essential fats—to function *optimally* and maintain good health. And the cold hard fact is that most of us are not getting what we need for our short- and long-term health—not by a very long shot. Here's why:

- ✔ We eat overly processed foods and fast foods that have been stripped of their original nutrient content.

- ✔ We eat foods grown in nutrient-depleted soils. Therefore, the vegetables, grains, and fruits grown in these fields aren't as healthful as they once were.

- ✔ We lead stressful lifestyles that increase our bodies' demand for certain nutrients.

With all this in mind, it's not hard to understand why nutritional deficiencies are so widespread. Think about this: Statistics show that one out of every eight of us will get cancer. One out of five will develop heart disease. And another one out of four will get diabetes. It could happen to you or me next year, next month, or even *tomorrow.*

But, more and more, research shows that we have the power to prevent or promote these terrible and debilitating diseases simply by what we put into our bodies.

Commandment #10: Drink lots of water.

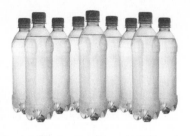

Another very important key to getting a flat belly is remembering to drink *lots* of water. How much? Before each of your five mini-meals during the day, drink 12 ounces of pure, fresh water—that's the same amount of fluid found in the average soft drink can. Then drink *another* 12 ounces of water with your meal. Because you will be eating five mini-meals each day on the *Belly Fat Free* Program, that's a minimum of 10 glasses of water each and every day.

Many people think drinking water will make them look bloated. But I assure you the exact opposite is true. Most men and women are actually in a constant state of mild dehydration, so their bodies hoard water like a squirrel stores acorns for winter. If you begin drinking an increased amount of water (about 10 glasses) for a few days, your body will naturally release excess water weight and you'll become less bloated and lighter.

Water helps flush out toxins that can be released when fat is burned for energy and is involved in our body's metabolic functions. Another important thing to keep in mind is that water makes up 75 percent of muscle tissue. Not to mention that it plays a key role in burning stored fat as fuel. So you may not lose fat as easily if you aren't properly hydrated. (Get my drift?)

> Being dehydrated by as little as 1 or 2 percent of your body weight can impair both mental and physical functions—including fat burning.

Did you know that being dehydrated by as little as 1 or 2 percent of your body weight can impair both mental and physical functions? That includes burning body fat, by the way. (Fatigue and weakness can result from not drinking enough water as well.) I suggest carrying water with you while you work, play, and exercise—try to get in the habit of sipping it throughout the day.

The key is to drink water even when you're *not* thirsty, because by the time your body clues you in, you're already too low. So put away those diet soft drinks and sugar-filled fruit juices. Instead, replenish your body with lots of pure water.

Commandment #11:
Build your confidence daily.

To be successful, it's *vital* to feed your confidence and to improve your self-image each and every day. This is *just* as important as following my eating and activity tips. (For details, review Chapter 3.)

Make no mistake, **none of us can outperform our self-images.** Building confidence is the *real* secret behind *Belly Fat Free*.

Commandment #12:
Develop coping skills.

While following BFF you *will* need to overcome adversity. You *will* have setbacks. After all, life is not always a bed of roses, and things come up that we can't anticipate. But you can prepare for certain events ahead of time. Here are some suggestions:

1. Make large amounts of great-tasting healthy food and freeze them. This way you won't turn to junk food when you're on the run. See my *Belly Fat Free Cookbook,* available at BellyFatFree.com/Cookbook, for recipes.

2. Carry these pre-prepared meals with you to work in a cooler.

3. Carry a meal replacement drink mix or nutrition bar with you for emergencies. The Belly Fat Free Smoothies™ and Belly Fat Free Nutrition Bars™ are good choices.

4. Empty all junk food from your refrigerator and pantry and replace it with healthful foods. (See Chapter 7 for full details.)

5. When you can't control a craving, opt for alternate choices instead of the real deal. Instead of a candy bar enjoy a piece or two of a chocolate bar with a 70% to 80% cocoa content. Instead of sneaking a super-sized soft drink for that caffeine high, have some green tea, or naturally flavored warm teas (without sugar or artificial sweeteners), which may still contain caffeine but in much smaller amounts. Or, have a soft drink alternative like Zevia which can be found at Whole Foods. For all my product choices visit BellyFatFree.com/GoodBad. Just do your best to avoid those nasty obesity additives.

6. Get an exercise bench, a few dumbbells, and a used exercise bike for your home or office so you don't skip workouts.

7. If you work out at a health club, keep an extra set of workout clothes in your car so you don't skip the gym because you forgot to bring them.

8. Constantly reread your answers to the questions from the BFF Confidence Booster in Chapter 3. This will keep you inspired and on track.

When cravings get out of control between meals, drink a large glass of water and do some mild exercise or stress-relieving activities (stretching, deep breathing, meditation). Believe it or not, I also find that brushing my teeth helps settle cravings as well.

Commandment #13:
Find a role model and create a support system.

Here's a secret: If you want to become a millionaire, hang out with millionaires. If you want to be a great parent, learn what great parents do by spending time with them. If you want to have a flat belly, find someone who lost belly fat (in a healthy manner) and model her process.

If you want to achieve something, there's almost always someone who has already accomplished it, and you can learn a tremendous amount from her experience. This person can help you shorten the learning curve and avoid a lot of potential mistakes along the way.

I'll do my best to be your BFF Coach both throughout this book and live at my weight loss coaching Web site, BellyFatFree.com. Here you can get instant access to weight loss tools like interactive forums, video weight loss classes, fat loss journals, and so much more. You can even get a weight loss buddy to help keep you accountable for your goals. (If you haven't visited this site, please do so now. You can interact with past Belly Fat Free Champions and people just like you from all over the world.)

Commandment #14:
Make yourself a priority.

"I don't have time." "I'm just too busy right now." These phrases account for the number-one excuse I hear from people who fail to lose weight and shape up. What they should really say is, "I don't *want* to make time right now."

The fact of the matter is that getting slim and trim doesn't take time, it *makes* time. How? I know from personal experience that excess weight slows you down, zaps your energy levels, and halts productivity. Having enough energy is always a big problem. But losing weight invigorates and energizes the body and mind.

We both know there will never be a perfect time to get going. You're always going to be busy. And, if you wait for that perfect time to come…well, you'll be waiting forever. So why not get going today?

And if you *still* think you're too busy, here are a few time-saving tips to help you make time for this program:

✔ *Limit TV time.* Statistics say the average American watches 30 hours of television per week. That means chances are you can save a *lot* of time by limiting your television viewing to a few shows or movies per week. Or if you just can't miss your favorite show, try exercising while you watch it. You can lift weights or ride a stationary bike and kill two birds with one stone.

✔ *Turn off the phone and Internet.* I see people wasting hour upon hour chatting away on cell phones, house phones, and instant messenger. Again, I suggest multitasking whenever possible—talk and walk if need be. The same goes for texting, online surfing, and e-mailing. Why write a 30-minute e-mail when a five-minute phone call will do?

✔ *Exercise first thing in the morning.* Otherwise, life often gets in the way and it never gets done. Treat yourself to 15 to 30 minutes of "you time" at sunrise by getting your heart pumping and starting the day off right.

✔ *Install time blocking.* This simply means setting time aside that is specifically dedicated to losing weight during your day. Maybe it's at 5:30 a.m. or 11 p.m. It doesn't matter as long as it's set in stone.

✔ *Set up your home fitness center.* You don't need fancy equipment to get slim—a few dumbbells, an exercise bench, and a stationary bike will do the trick. (Check out eBay.com or a used sporting goods store for inexpensive items.) We'll talk about what equipment you need in Chapter 9. Keep in mind that you can save a lot of time working out at home rather than driving to and from a crowded gym.

Commandment #15:
Focus on progress, not perfection.

Trust me…*everyone* falls off the weight loss wagon every now and then. The truth is, you just might lose control in a moment of weakness; it happens to all of us. But when it does, true champions immediately get back in the saddle. Those without the proper mindset figure they've already screwed up, so they may as well *really* screw up and continue gorging. That's akin to getting a flat tire on your car and deciding you may as well slash the other three tires because one is already flat.

BFF Assignment #6 ☐
Find 30 Minutes In Your Day

Using the time-saving tips mentioned in Commandment 14, figure out where you can carve 30 minutes out of each day just for you. You'll use this time to prepare healthier foods, be more active, and to put the focus on yourself. Write your answer below:

_____

_____

Instead, if you *do* get off track, simply get back on your program as soon as humanly possible. Perfection is a myth. Nothing is perfect. You should focus on progress and celebrate your daily accomplishments.

So there you have it, your BFF Commandments. Follow them and your chances for success will dramatically increase. Now it's time to get to the specifics of the program—what to eat and when. It all starts in the next chapter.

The 15 BFF Commandments

1. Reduce sugar intake.

2. Eat more fiber.

3. Replenish your good bacteria.

4. Eat tasty foods every three hours.

5. Balanced meals are the key to your success.

6. Count cups. Not calories.

7. Move your body.

8. Lock up your scale.

9. Only use scientifically backed weight loss supplements.

10. Drink lots of water.

11. Build your confidence daily.

12. Develop coping skills.

13. Find a role model and create a support system.

14. Make yourself a priority.

15. Focus on progress, not perfection.

BFF Success Story
Marie: Grandma Loses Weight After 40 Years of Struggling

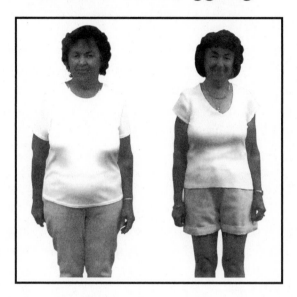

Once upon a time, Marie Seibel was overweight, out of shape, and all the way up to a size 18. Today she sports a fantastic new body and fits into a size four. At long last, she's happy, healthy, and living her ideal life.

This 64-year-old grandmother of five says, "I know the importance of good health. In August of 2000, just three weeks after his diagnosis, I lost my husband to a cancerous brain tumor. I was devastated. My husband was gone, and I was alone."

After giving herself time to grieve, Marie began her journey. She knew that in order to be successful, she had to focus on what she could control…not what she couldn't. She made a conscious decision to reclaim her health by first taking control of her thoughts and her body.

"Ask and you shall receive," Marie says, smiling. As soon as she decided she was going to transform her body, she learned about the Belly Fat Free Challenge from her sister. Marie remembers, "I read everything, and I was hooked. I was ready to win. The Challenge was just what I needed at that time in my life."

Choosing to make changes in life is rarely easy. Marie recalls, "For years and years I was addicted to beer. When I got thirsty, I drank beer. I knew it was bad for me, but I couldn't stop. Once I accepted the Challenge and read *Belly Fat Free*, it helped me eliminate my unhealthy addiction to beer. It was no longer going to have power over me."

Within the first week of beginning her program, Marie stopped drinking. "Now I keep ice-cold water in the refrigerator. Almost instantly I began feeling better. You know, before I learned about the importance of water, I used to think beer quenched my thirst. Now I know better. Alcohol only left me dehydrated and tired."

"In the past, I used drastic measures to lose weight. Nothing worked." Marie knew all the dieting, starving, and prescription diet drugs had to end. All it was accomplishing was making her unhealthy. Even more disappointing, the weight always came back. But this time, Marie was determined to succeed.

Furthermore, Marie had met someone special. She opened her heart again, found love, and soon after, she and Gary were married. "Gary is 23 years younger [than me], and that's one reason why it's important to look and feel good about myself. One day I got to thinking, 'I better get this weight off and trim down, so I look as good as—or even better than—all these young girls.'"

Marie's results were amazing. She wanted to lose about 15 pounds and have more energy, but not only did she meet her goal—she far exceeded it. **Marie lost an incredible 30 pounds**

and 27 ¾ inches. And she lost 7 pounds the very first week—all this without ever setting foot in a health club!

"I look at it like this: Your bicep does not know if you're lifting a brand-new, polished 12-pound dumbbell at Bally's or a 12-pound dumbbell in your basement. The only thing your bicep knows is that it's lifting 12 pounds. Just move. If you can get outside, walk. If not, do sit-ups, push-ups, fill old milk jugs with water and lift, walk in place while doing the dishes. Whatever you do, just don't sit there."

The pounds melted away and, almost daily, the scale moved downward. The more fat and inches Marie lost, the more self-esteem she gained. "Right away I could see and feel the results. I noticed an increase in energy. I knew I'd discovered something special."

Marie admits, "I keep that awful 'before' photo as my constant reminder of how far I have come. I have rebuilt my body, added years to my life, and greatly improved the quality of my life. I'm never going back." Marie also continues to coach and inspire other men and women at BellyFatFree.com. She says, "For 40 years I tried to lose the weight. Now that I finally learned how, it's my goal to help others avoid a lifetime of poor health and low self-esteem. I did it and I want to show them how, too."

CHAPTER 7

The BFF Eating Plan

We've all heard it before: You are what you eat. Well, guess what? It's absolutely true.

Picture a person who constantly eats unhealthy foods full of saturated fats, sugars, sodium, cholesterol, and preservatives (in other words, a typical American diet full of obesity additives). Are her muscles hidden under layers of body fat? Is she constantly tired? Does she get sick all the time or frequently feel "down in the dumps?"

Most likely, the answer to all these questions is "yes."

Now picture a healthy person—someone who nourishes her body with appropriate amounts of quality proteins, fruits, vegetables, complex carbohydrates, and "good" fats. What's different about her? A lot. Chances are she has muscle tone and plenty of energy. It's also likely that she's generally healthy and happy. In other words, her overall quality of life is far superior to that of someone who does not have good nutritional habits.

Think of it this way: Let's say you're building a house. But rather than using only top-notch supplies, you use inferior materials—rotten wood, cracked cement, faulty wiring, and leaky pipes.

141

You'll end up with a run-down, unsound, unattractive house, right?

Well, the same thing happens to your body when you feed it inferior food. You get a run-down body—one that is unhealthy and unattractive.

My point is this: The way our bodies look on the outside and feel on the inside is directly related to what we eat. Period. End of story. Simple, right?

Well, here's where it gets tricky. Most people don't know how to properly nourish their bodies. After all, this isn't the kind of information most folks actively research. And even if they *did* take the time to research how to eat right, they'd probably end up more confused than they were in the first place. It seems every "expert" has his own overly complicated opinion.

Are you ready for the good news? *It doesn't have to be this way.* Proper nutrition isn't that complicated. In fact, it can be boiled down to a few very simple, easy-to-follow strategies.

And I'd like to share those with you now.

Oh…one more thing. Please don't make the mistake of thinking proper nutrition should take a back seat to exercise. The truth is, the two go hand in hand. Think of them like wheels on a bicycle; just one won't get you where you want to go.

That said, make no mistake—the first step to creating a Belly Fat Free body is to begin nourishing yourself with the nutrients you need from the inside out. Keep in mind that virtually *every* cell in your body is replaced each and every year. And where do you think your body gets the building blocks to replace each cell? That's right, food. So if you want a better body, you have to consume better building blocks.

With all that in mind, here are (drum roll, please!) my BFF Eating Secrets.

Eat All Day Long

My students often ask me what my number one tip is for shedding unwanted and unattractive belly fat while increasing muscle tone, energy, and overall health.

My response is always, "Eat every three hours for a total of five mini-meals throughout the day."

Why is this important? Well, the answer may surprise you. You see, when you only eat a few meals a day, your body will begin to naturally slow down your metabolism and inhibit (reduce) fat burning. Instead, your body will begin to burn your muscle tissue as an energy source.

Here's why that's bad: The amount of muscle you have plays a big role in how many calories you burn throughout the day. For example, look at a big NFL football player who has a great deal of muscle mass. If you have seen one of these guys eat—or if you've seen a growing teenage boy eat—you know that he can eat a lot of food without gaining a lot of fat. He may eat an entire large pizza in one sitting and *still* be hungry. This is one of the benefits to having more muscle...you can eat more without gaining more.

> One of the benefits to having more muscle is that you can eat more without gaining more.

Your body burns approximately 50 extra calories for every pound of muscle you have. That's why it is vitally important to preserve and build your muscle while decreasing your fat levels. (Most dieters don't focus on building muscle while losing weight,

Case in Point

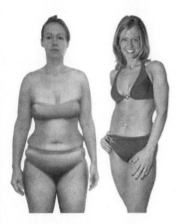

Tina White, a former BFF Champion, put on six pounds of lean, attractive muscle during her transformation. As I just mentioned, each pound of muscle burns about 50 extra calories per day. So when Tina added six pounds of muscle, her body naturally burned 300 extra calories per day whether she exercised or not.

Now consider this: 300 additional calories per day equals 2,100 additional calories per week, and 8,400 additional calories per month. When you think about it this way and bear in mind that one pound of fat contains 3,500 calories, you will soon realize that Tina will naturally burn the calorie equivalent of about two-and-a-half pounds of fat per month...just to support her increase in muscle. This all means that Tina will burn the calorie equivalent of 31 pounds of fat per year just by adding six pounds of lean, attractive muscle to her frame!

Tina can now eat more *and* still maintain or even lose weight. Amazing!

so half of the weight they lose is muscle. This is a very bad thing because it kills your metabolism.)

This is why I strongly encourage you to take part in the BFF Resistance Routine, featured in Chapter 9. Resistance training is a great way to increase your lean muscle mass while burning additional calories.

Burning fat and preserving muscle—which keeps your metabolism humming along—is just one benefit of eating every three hours. Which leads us to an interesting question: Why in the world does your body begin to shut down fat burning and increase muscle burning after just three hours or so?

You see, again, back in the "caveman days" our ancestors lived by feast or famine. When food was plentiful they would gorge themselves and subsequently accumulate a great deal of additional body fat. But in times when food was scarce, their bodies would naturally conserve the most calorie-dense energy source they had—which was body fat—and begin burning muscle instead. So, in a nutshell, when your body isn't receiving a constant supply of food it will begin to sabotage your weight loss efforts by switching from fat-burning to muscle-burning mode, slowing down your metabolism in the process.

A large amount of scientific research backs up the positive effects of eating frequently. In fact, one of my favorite studies shows that two groups of individuals, given the same amount of calories over the same period of time, ended up achieving different weight loss results. You guessed it! The group who ate frequent meals (every three hours) actually ended up losing much more weight than the group who ate only three meals per day even though they were consuming an *identical* number of calories.

How is this possible? Well, the answer is very exciting. Every time you eat a meal your body must use calories to digest and process the food so your metabolism increases. Eat more often and you boost your metabolism more often. Makes sense, right? Well, the more complex a food is, the more calories your body uses to digest and process it. Be sure to keep that in mind the next time you reach for a highly processed food like most cereals, baked goods, soft drinks, and desserts.

A Calorie is Not a Calorie

Make no mistake, some foods will increase your metabolism, while others won't affect your metabolism much at all. This is precisely why some of those "point systems" that tell you to eat whatever you want as long as you don't exceed your daily allotted points are seriously flawed diet plans.

Calories from different types of food act very differently once in your body. Food scientists and nutritionists refer to this as the thermic effect of food. Here's an example: Your metabolic rate (or metabolism) will increase by approximately 5 percent in response to eating fats. This means that for every 100 calories of fat you eat, your body will burn five of its own calories to digest and process them.

When you eat carbohydrates, your metabolic rate will increase by approximately 10 percent (less for refined carbs like sugar). This means your body uses 10 calories to digest and use 100 calories of carbs. Protein has the highest thermic effect of all foods, increasing your metabolism by approximately 20 percent. Protein is a very complex nutrient, so for every 100 calories of protein you eat, your body will use about 20 calories to digest and process them. This means you're only netting about 80 calories for every 100 calories you eat of protein. Pretty cool, huh?

All of this explains why complex, unprocessed natural foods like lean meats, low-fat dairy, vegetables, and whole grains are good choices—your body uses more calories to digest them. Simple foods like sugars and processed white carbohydrates, on the other hand, are already broken down, so your body doesn't have to use as many calories to digest them. This is thanks to our good friends the food manufacturers, who have already done the processing for you. This is one of the reasons it's important to stay away from processed foods (like white breads, cereals, pastas, soft drinks, and various sugar-filled items) if you're interested in losing body fat. (While we're on the subject, another big reason to avoid them is that they absorb and convert to fat quickly.)

I'm not suggesting that you eat nothing but protein in an attempt to increase your metabolism. No, not at all. But what I *am* suggesting is that you eat balanced mini-meals throughout the day that include protein, carbs, and a smaller amount of good fat (more on this in a minute).

The bottom line is this: Eating a balanced mini-meal every three hours throughout the day will boost your body's natural metabolism for a few hours every time you eat. Then it will return to normal. So what happens if you wait hours and hours to eat again? That's right, your metabolism will remain "normal" until you feed it—or worse, it will come to a screeching halt. By eating every three hours, you keep your calorie-burning metabolism humming along at full speed, all day long.

Are you starting to see why eating every three hours is of the utmost importance for those who want fast results?

Other Benefits to Eating Every Three Hours

Yep, there's more! As if boosting your metabolism wasn't enough, these daily mini-meals will also increase your energy levels and balance your mood because your blood sugar levels are stabilized and your brain and body are receiving a constant supply of nutrients to help them stay sharp and energized.

This is a *huge* bonus because you can harness this mental energy and stability to accomplish those dreams that have been sitting on the back burner for years. And you can use this newfound physical energy to have more intense and productive workouts (or you can begin working out in the first place—hint, hint).

Suppressing Appetite and Cravings

When my students first hear about these mini-meals, many of them look at me in shock and are scared they'll begin to gain weight rather than lose it. I promise you, this could not be further from the truth. By eating a mini-meal every three hours, you will not only increase your metabolism, but you will also suppress your appetite—especially if you are combining the *right* types of foods (more on this shortly).

It works like this: After you eat a highly "processed" meal, your blood sugar level quickly rises. A surge of fat-storing insulin is released from your pancreas to store this blood sugar as body fat. As a result, your blood sugar levels then decrease dramatically, causing your energy levels to crash. Soon, you feel tired, hungry, and are hit with a tidal wave of cravings.

Millions of Americans experience this crash and burn cycle every hour of every day. It's a shame that they don't realize how easy it is to boost their energy levels and mood while simultaneously decreasing hunger and cravings, simply by controlling how they time their food intake.

I find it very interesting that drug companies are desperately trying to come up with a way to control leptin, that hormone we discussed in Chapter 4. Why? Because this particular hormone is released by fat cells and plays a big role in controlling your hunger and cravings. Studies indicate that you can actually control leptin levels yourself—without a drug—by eating frequent unprocessed meals. Why pay money for a medication when you can accomplish the same results by eating five mini-meals per day?

Another reason I love to eat every three hours is because I am not as apt to overeat. It's simple. After eating a mini-meal I think to myself, "I don't need to eat any more because, after all, I'm going to be eating again in just three hours. Why stuff myself now?" As a result, most people's stomachs shrink back to normal size, and they begin to get full faster and stay full longer.

Furthermore, I also like to eat every three hours because… well, I like to eat! It's no secret that I had an addiction to certain foods. The chemicals in these foods used to control my life—they certainly controlled my overweight body. But when I began to eat frequently I broke that addiction. Now I have control over my food…and so can you.

Belly Fat Buster

Need another reason to eat every three hours?

Well, here you go. Your body has a stress hormone called cortisol. This hormone is associated with causing excess belly fat; the more cortisol you have, the more belly fat you typically gain. Now get this: The *New England Journal of Medicine* published a study showing that individuals who consumed mini-meals spaced three hours apart actually *decreased* their cortisol levels by 17 percent compared to those who ate the same amount of food in three meals per day.

And here's some even better news. This cortisol-blunting effect occurred in just 14 days. So if you want to take control of your body's cortisol levels, there's no need to take an expensive supplement (some of which could cost you hundreds of dollars a month). Simply start eating a small mini-meal every three hours to reduce cortisol up to 17 percent on your own.

Those are just a few of the benefits to eating five mini-meals a day, three hours apart. Now I have to admit, I've found that when my clients begin eating this way it feels very unnatural to them in the beginning. You see, as Americans, most of us have stretched our stomachs out to the point where we just don't feel satisfied unless we're gorging on a huge calorie-laden meal every chance we get.

So when you begin eating a mini-meal every three hours you may not feel completely full after each meal. But that will quickly change. The truth is, after just a few days of eating five mini-meals, your stomach will naturally begin to shrink in size, and the small mini-meals will leave you feeling full, satisfied, light, and energetic. (Most of you can forget about gastric bypass surgeries to shrink your stomach. Eating small, frequent, balanced meals—that don't contain obesity additives—can do the same thing…naturally.)

Make no mistake, if you do *nothing* else in this program but begin to eat balanced mini-meals, spaced three hours apart throughout the day, you are going to make a great change in your body. However, if you incorporate all of the suggestions in this chapter, you will quickly transform your body in as little as 12 weeks.

The BFF Eating Schedule

Now that we've talked about spreading out smaller meals throughout the course of the day, I want to talk about your daily eating schedule in its entirety.

I think the best way to start is by giving you an example of what I do. Here goes: I typically get up at 6 a.m. and get my 30 minutes of daily exercise accomplished right off the bat. By the way, studies show you can burn fat up to *300 percent* faster by exercising first thing in the morning on an empty stomach. Because your blood sugar levels are naturally lower, your body will be more likely to burn stored body fat instead of sugar from the foods you recently ate. What's more, exercise calms me and gives me peace of mind and clarity for the rest of the day. It's a scientific fact that exercise fights stress.

After my exercise, I take the next 30 minutes to get ready for my day—I take a shower, brush my teeth, comb my hair—that sort of stuff. This gives my body an extra 30 minutes to continue to burn stored body fat at an accelerated rate after exercise.

> Studies show you can burn fat up to *300 percent* faster by exercising first thing in the morning on an empty stomach.

I then have my first mini-meal of the day at 7 a.m. My next mini-meal will be at 10 a.m., then 1 p.m., 4 p.m., and my last at 7 p.m.

Now seems like the perfect time to fill you in on another big secret to my Belly Fat Free Eating Plan—**don't eat right before going to bed.**

I try to go to bed around 10 p.m. so I get in my eight hours of sleep per night, which is *vitally important* to anyone interested in zapping belly fat, building muscle, and improving his or her health. That's why my last meal of the night is typically at 7 p.m.—three hours before bedtime.

Now I have to admit, some nights I'm hungry even after my 7 p.m. meal, so I *may* sneak in a sixth mini-meal consisting of a Belly Fat Free Smoothie, half a turkey sandwich, or a low-sugar yogurt. (I like the Oikos Greek Yogurt brand without artificial sweeteners. I pour a packet of truvia™ natural sweetener into it for added sweetness.) There is no problem with having this sixth mini-meal *if you really need it.* After all, it's much better than having a large meal during the day and then a second huge pig-out session right before bed.

The problem with eating just before bedtime is, of course, you're not active while you sleep. So any food you eat just before bed is digested and stored during the night. Additionally, you want your body's main nighttime focus to be on repairing and replenishing your body cells, like, for instance, those cells found in your immune system. But if you go to bed with a large amount of food in your digestive system, your body will be forced to deal with this food instead of focusing all of its efforts on healing and building your body. Going to bed on a full stomach can also disrupt your natural sleep cycle so that you do not experience a deep, sound sleep.

Here's what I want you to take away from all this in just a couple of sentences: Do your best to stop eating three hours before bedtime. If you do need a snack, make sure it's one that contains both protein and healthy carbs, not a Big Mac and fries.

Recommended BFF Foods

By now you understand the importance of timing your food by eating a mini-meal every three hours. But you're probably confused about what foods to eat, how much to eat, and how to combine your foods for maximum fat loss. So, let's cover those topics now, beginning with my Recommended BFF Foods.

To make things simple, I've divided my Belly Fat Free Food Groups not by categories like meats, dairy, grains, fruits, and vegetables, but rather by what macronutrient each food *primarily* contains. A macronutrient is either a protein, a carbohydrate, or a fat. (Alcohol can also be considered a macronutrient—but it's not a necessary food group unless you're in a college fraternity.)

I also separate carbohydrates into two subgroups: *energy carbs* and *color carbs.* I do this because energy carbs contain more calories per cup than color carbs do. For example, a cup of potatoes can easily contain double the calories of a cup of broccoli. Sure, they both contain primarily carbohydrates, but one is much more calorie dense then the other.

Let's kick things off by talking about proteins.

Proteins

Proteins are primarily used as our bodies' building blocks. They are most abundant in animal products—lean meats, egg whites, and low-fat cottage cheese are great protein sources. (Protein is also found, to a lesser degree, in beans, nuts, and various grains for you vegetarians out there.) Proteins are found in every cell in our bodies. Our muscles, hair, skin, nails, hormones, and blood all contain protein. And protein is extremely important both to our overall immunity and health.

Protein is also an ***extremely*** important (but often overlooked) fat-loss nutrient. Why? Proteins (along with resistance exercise) actually help your body change shape by adding muscle and increasing your metabolism. Remember, the point isn't just to lose weight. *The point is to lose fat, and increase muscle.*

Carbohydrates

Our bodies primarily use carbohydrates as an energy source. Carbohydrates come from plants (or trees) that store starch, sugar, and fiber in grains, fruits, and vegetables.

Carbohydrates often get a bad rap, which is a shame because carbs are your body's preferred source of fuel. Some cells (like your brain and blood cells, for example) are very limited in the types of energy they can use, with a strong preference for simple carbohydrates. If you've ever been on a no-carb diet and experienced that lightheaded, queasy, hit-the-wall feeling, you know what I'm talking about.

> Carbohydrates often get a bad rap, which is a shame because carbs are your body's preferred source of fuel.

Recommended BFF Protein -Rich Foods

- Anchovies
- Bass
- Beef (extra-lean)
- Bluefish
- Buffalo
- Chicken breast
- Clams
- Cod
- Cornish hen
- Cottage cheese (1% or less)
- Crab
- Egg whites or egg substitutes
- Elk
- Flounder
- Grouper
- Haddock
- Halibut
- Herring
- Kefir
- Lamb loin
- Liver (beef, calf, or chicken)
- Lobster
- Mackerel
- Mahimahi
- Mussels
- Orange roughy
- Oysters
- Perch
- Pork (lean)
- Red snapper
- Roast (arm, chuck, or rump)
- Sablefish
- Salmon
- Sardines
- Scallops
- Scrod
- Shrimp
- Sirloin (ground)
- Sole
- Soy burger patty
- Steak (club, flank, round, sirloin, tenderloin, or T-bone filet; all fat trimmed)
- Swordfish
- Tilapia
- Trout
- Tuna (water-packed)
- Turkey bacon
- Turkey breast (lean ground or whole)
- Turkey sausage
- Veal
- Venison
- Whitefish
- Wild Alaskan salmon
- Yellow tail
- Yogurt (plain, 1% or less)

Recommended BFF Energy Carb Foods

- ✔ Bananas
- ✔ Barley
- ✔ Beans and lentils (dried)
- ✔ Bread (100% whole grain)
- ✔ Buckwheat
- ✔ Corn
- ✔ Corn tortillas
- ✔ Crackers (whole wheat like ak-mak, Kavli, Ryvita®, Wasa®)
- ✔ Cream of wheat (long-cooking—not instant)
- ✔ Oatmeal (whole grain, not instant)
- ✔ Pasta (100% whole grain)
- ✔ Potatoes (baking and sweet)
- ✔ Quinoa
- ✔ Rice (brown or wild)
- ✔ Yams

The key is to eat the *right* carbohydrates. Yes, there are right carbs and wrong carbs. Most simple carbs are the *wrong* carbs—in fact, they are one of the top obesity additives. They tend to be highly processed and stripped of their nutrients. Examples of foods that contain simple carbohydrates include soft drinks, candy bars, ice cream, donuts, cereals, and processed "white foods" like breads, pastas, and rice. (Remember, white foods are like white glue that keeps your belly fat locked in place.) Even though they may be tempting, these foods spike your blood sugar then send it crashing, zapping your energy and creating a breeding ground for cravings and body fat. Limit your intake of these to your splurge meals (which I'll explain in a minute).

Complex carbohydrates, on the other hand, have all the right stuff. These foods are the ones that provide your body with the energy it needs in a steady fashion (none of this blood sugar roller-coaster business), while also providing much-needed fiber and important vitamins and minerals to your body.

Recommended BFF
Color Carb Foods

- Apples
- Apricots
- Artichoke (including Jerusalem)
- Arugula
- Asparagus
- Bamboo shoot
- Beans (string)
- Bean sprouts
- Beets
- Berries
- Bok choy
- Broccoli
- Broccoli rabe
- Broccoli sprouts
- Brussels sprouts
- Cabbage
- Cantaloupe
- Cauliflower
- Celery
- Chard
- Cherries
- Cheese (fat-free)
- Chestnuts (water)
- Collard or mustard greens
- Cucumber
- Eggplant
- Escarole
- Garlic
- Grapefruit
- Grapes
- Green beans
- Honeydew melon
- Kale
- Kiwi
- Lemon
- Lettuce (endive or mixed greens)
- Lime
- Mango
- Milk (1% or less)
- Mushrooms
- Nectarines
- Okra
- Onions
- Oranges
- Papaya
- Peach
- Pear
- Peas (including snow peas)
- Pea pods
- Peppers (bell or hot)
- Pineapple
- Plums
- Prunes
- Radish
- Rhubarb
- Rutabaga
- Spinach
- Squash (yellow)
- Tangerine
- Tomato
- Turnip
- Watermelon
- Yogurt (low-sugar)
- Zucchini

Complex carbohydrates can be further broken down into what I like to call energy carbs and color carbs. Energy carbs are nutrient-dense turbo chargers. Whole grains and starchy foods are great examples of energy carbs. If you're looking for power and vitality, these little gems are your best bet.

Color carbs contain rich sources of fiber, but their real claim to fame is that they provide phytonutrients, important chemicals found in plants that support a variety of health functions. A specific family of phytonutrients called anthocyanins is responsible for compounds that give fruits and veggies their vibrant color.

Here's the real kicker, though—anthocyanins also pack a powerful antioxidant punch. Different color pigments carry different health benefits. For example, lutein, an important nutrient for eye health, is found in yellow-green vegetables such as corn and peas. Lycopene, found in tomatoes, is not only responsible for their red color but also supports prostate health. Orange carotenoids found

Got Milk?

You're probably wondering where dairy products fall on these lists. Are they proteins, energy carbs, or color carbs? The answer is ... it depends. Cottage cheese is primarily protein, so it falls in the protein category. Skim milk, yogurt, and fat-free (or low-fat) cheeses are really a combination of protein and carb with at least twice as many carbs on average. For simplicity's sake, we're going to add these items to the color carb list. Remember, we're classifying food based on what it's primarily made up of—protein, energy carbs, color carbs, or fats. There's no need to make eating more complicated than it needs to be. This keeps it simple.

in carrots, pumpkins, and apricots have been found to enhance immune system function. Sulphorapane gives broccoli and brussels sprouts their green color, and it also happens to be a potent weapon against cancer. And reddish-purple anthocyanins, found in blueberries, blackberries, and plums, pump up circulation and protect the brain.

Fats

Our bodies use fats as sources for long-term energy. Fats are also used to build hormones and body cells. Essential fats—often called good fats or omega fats—are fats that our bodies can't produce on their own; we need to get them from the foods we eat. The problem is that most of the good fats naturally found in our food supply are destroyed during processing and cooking. These special good fats are found in every cell of the body and are important because they play a role in virtually every body function, including hormone production and inflammation regulation. Essential fats also help your body burn stored body fat by affecting the balance of the hormones insulin and glucagon (insulin stores fats and glucagon signals the body to burn it).

Quality sources of good fats include oils such as flax, olive, and coconut. Good fats are also found in seafood sources such

Recommended BFF Fat Foods

- ✔ Almonds
- ✔ Avocados
- ✔ Canola oil
- ✔ Flax oil
- ✔ Olive oil
- ✔ Pumpkin seed oil

- ✔ Salmon (also a protein source)
- ✔ Sunflower oil
- ✔ Tuna (also a protein source)
- ✔ Walnuts

What You Need to Know About Fat

Although your body does require fat, it's imperative to bear in mind that fat is a very calorie-dense macronutrient that you definitely don't want to overeat—especially the saturated versions.

Let's say I'm thinking about getting a bag of reduced-fat cheddar cheese. That's a good choice, right? After all, cheese is full of calcium *and* it's reduced-fat. That means it's a good choice, right?

Sort of.

When you check out the food label you'll see that out of 80 total calories per serving (which is only ¼ cup—most people use ¼ cup on just one taco), 60 calories are from fat. That means that this food is 75 percent fat by calories.

Here's a formula for figuring out what you're *really* looking at when it comes to fat.

Total fat calories ÷ Total calories = % of calories from fat

So, in this case, you have 60 fat calories ÷ 80 total calories for a total of 0.75 or 75 percent fat. Kind of confusing, huh? Make no mistake, the food manufacturers like it this way. They don't want us to know how much fat they're sneaking into our food. After all, if we knew, we may make a different (better) choice.

Should you bring a calculator to the grocery store with you? Sure, why not? After all, it is your body and health we're talking about here.

as salmon and tuna, as well as in avocados and nuts like walnuts and almonds.

To make sure you're getting enough good fats in your diet (but not too many), I suggest adding two tablespoons of good oils to prepared foods each day, or having a serving of salmon or tuna (which also count as protein sources) three times a week. Alternatively, you may want to try ¼ cup of walnuts or almonds each day, or a tablespoon of organic peanut butter, or a high-quality essential fat supplement like Udo's Choice Oil Blend or Barlean's oil—try the Omega Swirl flavors. *

By the way, *be sure to avoid saturated fats as much as possible.* Saturated fats are primarily found in junk foods that are fried or highly processed, pasteurized whole milk dairy products, and fatty cuts of meat. Opt for low-fat versions whenever possible. (A notable exception is coconut oil, which is a healthier saturated fat that I recommend because it can actually help dieters lose weight. It's also one of the best cooking oils because it's very stable under high heat.)

---

* *Udo's Choice Oil Blend and Barlean's oils are available at most health food stores in the refrigerated section. In addition to providing a good fat source, they also do wonders for the health and appearance of hair and skin.*

BFF Assignment #7 ☐
Do Some Kitchen Math

Here's a little assignment: Grab your trusty calculator and go to your kitchen. Use the formula in the What You Need to Know About Fat section (page 159) and start putting those high school math skills to use. I think you'll be surprised that a lot of foods you thought were good for you are actually loaded with gobs of saturated fat. This fat is adding to your waistline and eroding your health.

Also, stay away from trans fats (often seen on food labels as partially hydrogenated oils). These man-made fats are toxic to the body and have been banned in much of Europe. Studies indicate these nasty fats increase the risk of a variety of cancers (turn to page 70 for a trans fat refresher). Check out your pantry, and you'll be surprised at how prominent these toxic fats are.

Other Food Suggestions

The foods listed in this chapter are highly recommended selections for the BFF Eating Plan, but they aren't the only healthy foods you can include in your new healthy eating habits. For a list of specific BFF good and bad food products be sure to check out BellyFatFree.com/GoodBad.

Don't forget that food choices aren't the only important factor to consider. Food preparation is just as important. Avoid foods that are fried or drenched in fatty sauces. Instead, opt for natural,

Fresh Herbs and Spices to Liven Up Your Food

✔ Anise	✔ Cinnamon	✔ Nutmeg
✔ Allspice	(ground or	✔ Oregano
✔ Basil	sticks)	✔ Paprika
✔ Bay leaf	✔ Cloves	✔ Parsley
✔ Caraway	✔ Coriander	✔ Peppercorns
✔ Cardamom	✔ Cumin	✔ Rosemary
✔ Cayenne	✔ Dill	✔ Sage
✔ Celery seed	✔ Fennel	✔ Saffron
✔ Chili flakes	✔ Garlic	✔ Savory
✔ Chives	✔ Ginger	✔ Tarragon
✔ Chervil	✔ Lemon balm	✔ Turmeric
✔ Cilantro	✔ Marjoram	✔ Thyme
	✔ Mint	✔ Vanilla bean

healthful foods that are steamed, grilled, broiled, or baked. The Herbs and Spices box on the previous page provides a few ideas for maximizing flavor while keeping it healthy. The best of both worlds!

BFF Cup Method™

I don't know about you, but I'm not a big fan of counting calories. It can be an all-day affair! Having said that, I *do* think reviewing food labels and knowing what's in your food is extremely important.

So that I don't have to measure, weigh, and count every piece of food that goes into my mouth, I often follow the BFF Cup Method. This is a very simple approach to eating that will ensure you're combining your foods properly to slow digestion, reduce fat storage, and to transform your body over the next 12 weeks. (Note: The Cup Method is optional. You can lose that belly just by consuming foods that don't contain addicting and calorie-dense obesity additives. Some of my top students have done this with amazing results.)

Here's how it works in three easy steps:

1. Choose ½ cup of a recommended Belly Fat Free Protein-Rich Food for each of your five daily mini-meals.

2. For three of your five mini-meals, add in one cup of a recommended Belly Fat Free Energy Carb.

3. For the other two of your five mini-meals, add in one cup of a recommended Belly Fat Free Color Carb.

And for good measure, here it is again in a slightly different way: You will have half a cup of protein and one cup of an energy carb for three of your five daily mini-meals. For the other two meals of the day, you will have half a cup of protein and one cup of a color carb. Your daily eating plan may look something like this:

- ✔ **Meal #1** (7 a.m.): ½ cup protein with one cup color carb
- ✔ **Meal #2** (10 a.m.): ½ cup protein with one cup energy carb
- ✔ **Meal #3** (1 p.m.): ½ cup protein with one cup energy carb
- ✔ **Meal #4** (4 p.m.): ½ cup protein with one cup color carb
- ✔ **Meal #5** (7 p.m.): ½ cup protein with one cup energy carb

Note: This amount of food works great if you weigh 200 pounds or less. If you weigh more than 200 pounds, please make the following adjustments:

- ✔ 201 to 250 pounds — Increase your carb intake to one and one-half cups per mini-meal.

- ✔ 251 to 300 pounds — Increase your carb intake to two cups per mini-meal.

- ✔ 301 pounds or more — Increase your carb intake to two cups per mini-meal, and add a sixth meal each day containing half a cup of protein and two cups of an energy carb.

Don't forget to adjust your food as your weight drops. Also, if you're eating a carbohydrate source that contains both color and energy carbs together (rice with cranberries, for example), always count it as an energy carb selection.

The Belly Fat Free Cup Method is a very simple, low-maintenance way to ensure you're getting the right amount of calories per day in the proper proportions of proteins, carbohydrates, and fats.

Remember, in the BFF Cup Method, a cup is a level cup. A half-cup is a level half-cup. That's it. Simple. Easy. No room for error. Now all you have to do is choose from the BFF Recommended Foods for each meal, eat them in the recommended amounts, and you're on your way to weight loss success. Simple!

By the way, the best way to avoid missing one of your five daily mini-meals is to always bring one with you everywhere you go. I make sure to have one quarter cup of almonds and an apple or banana with me at all times. I also always have a Belly Fat Free Bar or Smoothie on hand. This keeps me on track, and I never get hungry.

One more tip for now: If you're still hungry after one of your mini-meals—which is quite possible, especially when you first begin the program—and you can't wait until your next meal three hours later, just add another half-cup protein or one cup of a color carb to your mini-meal. It's better to increase your food intake initially than to fail before you even get going.

BFF Splurge Meals

We all have cravings now and then. If you feel one coming on for something really bad like pizza, cookies, or a hot fudge sundae, there's an ace in the hole for you—your weekly *splurge meals.* During these meals, you can eat anything you want as long as it doesn't exceed your mini-meal limit of one and one-half cups of total food (for those under 200 pounds; if you're 201 pounds or more, see page 163 and adjust accordingly).

And when I say you can eat anything, I mean *anything.* Have a piece of pan pizza. Gobble down a hamburger. Enjoy some hot, salty French fries or even a piece of cheesecake. Indulge in whatever you want. And, most importantly, enjoy it!

Why a Splurge Meal?

I recommend splurge meals because you're only setting yourself up for failure if you start an eating program that forbids you from ever eating your very favorite foods. It's just not realistic. Besides, splurging will settle those deep-seated psychological cravings that often emerge in an attempt to destroy your efforts just as you're starting to make some progress.

You wanna know something else? These splurge meals can actually kick start your metabolism too. Mixing up a lower-calorie eating plan with a quick burst of calories can fool your body into keeping its metabolism revving full-speed ahead.

Here are a couple more details about the Belly Fat Free Splurge Meal option:

1. During the first week of your 12-week program, you will have *three* splurge meals throughout the week. This will help wean you off the obesity additives and break the addiction.

2. Beginning your second week, the number of splurge meals per week will drop down to *two*.

Make sure to use these splurge meals wisely and plan for them ahead of time. For example, use a splurge meal when you are going out to eat with friends or for a special celebration. And don't forget, after the splurge meal (unless it's your last meal of the day), you're still going to be eating again three hours later. Finally, be sure not to eat more than the prescribed amount of total food based on your weight.

> Mixing up a lower-calorie eating plan with a quick burst of calories can fool your body into keeping its metabolism revving full-speed ahead.

Do you have to include these splurge meals? Nope. In fact, if you're the type of person who can't control herself after eating certain addictive foods—like French fries, ice cream, pie, cake, or chips—then I encourage you to skip these splurge meals entirely. They are not mandatory.

Some people (like me) have a hard time getting back on track after eating anything with obesity additives in it—especially sugar.

If you're this type of person (and you know who you are), then I encourage you to stay away from foods that cause you to fall off the wagon.

One more thing about splurge meals: *do not have these splurge foods in your home.* Make a point of leaving your house to indulge. Your home needs to be a safe, healthy environment free from "toxic waste" and temptation.

After you eat a splurge meal, take a moment to take stock of how you feel for the next few hours. If you eat foods with obesity additives in them, take note of their power to alter your mood—just like a drug. Many of my students report feeling nauseous and lightheaded (even sick) after reintroducing these artificial food substances back into their bodies. Other men and women also report a surge of hunger and cravings.

The Calorie Counter's Corner

If you're one of those people who just loves to count calories and you can't follow a program without doing so, my suggestion is to take your current body weight times the number eight. This will give you a rough estimate of how many calories you should consume over the course of a day to lose weight.

Body weight x 8 = Maximum daily calories to lose weight

Of course, always remember that exercise will burn additional calories.

To take it a step further, to plan your five mini-meals, just take the number of daily calories and divide that number by five. Here's how this little equation works for me: I currently weigh 170 pounds. 170 x 8 = 1,360 calories per day. 1,360 ÷ 5 = 272 calories per mini-meal.

If you want to break it down even further, try to follow a plan that is 30 percent protein, 45 percent carbs, and 25 percent good fat. When calculating your amounts, remember that protein and carbs contain four calories per gram, while fat contains nine calories per gram.

Whatever you do, be sure to include a protein source in each of your meals, along with a little fat and fiber. **Do not eat carbohydrates by themselves.** Proteins, fats, and fiber all slow down the digestion of your food and help lower the release of the fat-storing insulin.

Eating on the Run? No Problem.

I know, I know. If you're like a lot of my students you might be thinking, "It's going to be expensive and time consuming to prepare five mini-meals for myself every day." If so, you're not alone. In fact, most of my students say their three biggest obstacles to eating five mini-meals a day are:

✔ Healthy foods are too darn expensive and boring to eat.

✔ It's too time consuming to prepare five mini-meals each day.

✔ It's too confusing to know what foods to combine to create the best fat-burning effect.

Until recently, I couldn't agree more. I'd set aside two nights each week to cook all of my meals. Other times, when life was really busy, I'd post an ad and hire an inexpensive cook (or pay an eager friend or family member) to make healthy meals.

Once prepared, I'd keep some of this food in the refrigerator and freeze the rest in plastic containers. Each morning, I'd fill a small cooler with my frozen entrees and take them to work with me. Then when it was chow time, I'd reheat one in the microwave and enjoy.

This was pretty easy to do for lunch, but it became really difficult at other times of the day. Things would get hectic and I couldn't take the time to reheat food or sit down and eat. Before long I'd get so hungry I'd find myself frantically searching for the nearest vending machine for something…anything…to stuff in my face. It was almost always junk food, and I'd almost always eat too much of it to boot. (Ever do this?)

Then I discovered nutrition shakes and bars. These products can't totally replace whole food, but I can attest that they've made it infinitely easier to get that frequent infusion of healthy nutrients so critical to fat-loss success.

Imagine having a thick, rich, delicious milkshake that is perfectly balanced with the precise amounts of proteins, carbohydrates, vitamins, and minerals for one of your mini-meals. Here's the kicker: for less than 200 calories. Sound like a dieter's dream?

Actually it's a Belly Fat Free Smoothie—rich, creamy, and super easy to prepare. It takes just 60 seconds to create this smoothie (or

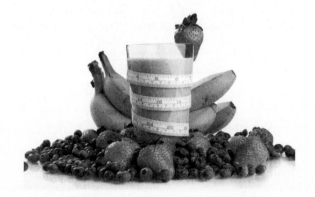

168   Belly Fat Free

mix it like pudding), and you've got a delicious, nutritious alternative to those fatty snacks that can add inches to your waist and thighs.

In each Belly Fat Free Smoothie you get one protein serving, one energy carb serving, and more vitamins and minerals then any color carb out there. These smoothies come in delicious flavors like Vanilla Cake Batter, Chocolate Cream, Chocolate Caramel, and Strawberry Banana Split.

BFF Smoothies contain a high-quality protein to help your body build muscle and to support an increased metabolism, plus a slow-release carbohydrate blend designed to slow digestion, which keeps energy levels up and reduces fat storage by controlling insulin levels. What's more, unlike other nutrition shakes, BFF Smoothies don't contain any obesity additives like hydrogenated oils/trans fats, high fructose corn syrup, artificial sweeteners, or large amounts of stripped carbohydrates.

These ingredients are big no-no's if you're trying to lose body fat and increase your health and energy levels. (If you see these ingredients in other products, run!) And in case you're wondering, Belly Fat Free Smoothies are 97 percent lactose free.

One BFF Smoothie contains:

- ✔ Only 140 calories
- ✔ 19 grams of high-quality whey protein isolate
- ✔ 9.5 grams of slow-absorbing Nutrim™
- ✔ Only two grams of sugar
- ✔ Three grams of good fats (you know, the ones that help burn fat)
- ✔ Three grams of healthy fiber
- ✔ 26 essential vitamins and minerals
- ✔ A special enzyme blend for easy, tummy-friendly digestion

Belly Fat Free Smoothies are like taking precise amounts of all the good stuff from food—the proteins, good carbs, good fats, fiber, and essential vitamins and minerals—and leaving out all the bad stuff. So you can feed your hunger and cravings while starving away the fat. (By the way, as I write this we are just putting the finishing touches on the new Belly Fat Free Bars that are based on the same delicious formula as the Belly Fat Free Smoothies. Our first flavors are Chocolate Mint Brownie and Oatmeal Raisin Cookie, and they taste just like they sound.)

Women and men across the country are achieving extraordinary results with Belly Fat Free Smoothies when used as part of a healthy eating and activity program. Unfortunately, the success stories you see in this book didn't have access to them, but you do! You can get BFF Bars and Smoothies at BellyFatFree.com.

You Gotta Love the Food You Eat

The bottom line is, if you don't enjoy the food you eat you won't be eating it for long. That's why you should make every attempt to feed yourself great-tasting foods every chance you get. Don't settle for bland, boring dishes that leave you physically full but mentally hungry.

Here's an example of a typical day's menu that I recommend for anyone following the BFF Eating Plan:

Meal #1: Strawberry Egg White Pancakes

4 egg whites (or the equivalent amount of egg substitute like Egg Beaters™)
4 tablespoons low-sugar strawberry preserves
½ cup old-fashioned oats
2 tablespoons 100% whole wheat pancake mix

Place all the ingredients in a blender and mix them well. Spray nonstick vegetable spray onto a medium-sized nonstick skillet and preheat the pan over medium heat. Pour the mixture into the skillet and cook the pancake for three to four minutes. Turn the pancake over and let it cook for an additional three minutes.

Serves four.

Meal #2: Belly Fat Free Vanilla Cake Batter Smoothie

Pour a scoop of BFF Smoothie mix into 8 ounces of cold water in a blender. Add a few ice cubes and blend at high speed for 30 seconds. Or you can use a "shaker bottle" to mix up a delicious smoothie without the mess or hassle of a blender.

Meal #3: My Favorite Lasagna

See recipe at the end of this chapter (page 185).

Meal #4: Low-Fat, Low-Sugar Yogurt

Meal #5: Grilled Chicken and Cranberry Rice

4 grilled, boneless, skinless chicken breasts
2 cups uncooked wild rice
1 16-ounce can low-fat chicken broth
1 cup dried cranberries or cherries

Grill the chicken breasts. In a saucepan, bring the broth to a boil and add rice. Reduce the heat to low. Cover the mixture and let it simmer until the rice has absorbed the broth. Toss in the dried cranberries and stir. Place a grilled chicken breast over a bed of cranberry rice. Refrigerate or freeze leftovers for later use.

Serves four.

You may be thinking this seems like a *lot* of food, but remember that each of these meals is actually quite small— between 200 and 350 calories if you follow the Cup Plan guidelines. It's important to change your perception of the *size* of a meal. Leaving the table a little hungry won't be so difficult if you know you're going to eat again in just three hours. Remember, after a week or so, your stomach will begin to "shrink" to a smaller size, and soon you will feel full and satisfied after each mini-meal.

Here's an example of a super convenient BFF Eating Plan for those hectic days on the run:

Quick Meal #1: Chocolate Raspberry Truffle Belly Fat Free Smoothie

Mix one Milk Chocolate Cream Belly Fat Free Smoothie and 8 ounces of water with a half cup frozen raspberries and three ice cubes. Blend the ingredients on high for 30 seconds.

Quick Meal #2: Cottage Cheese and Fruit

Measure a ½ cup of non-fat or 1% cottage cheese into a serving bowl. Add a cup of chilled, natural pineapple (or strawberries) with no sugar added.

Quick Meal #3: Belly Fat Free Chocolate Mint Brownie Nutrition Bar

Quick Meal #4: Turkey Sandwich

Pick up a six-inch turkey sandwich with mustard and veggies from Subway® or a similar restaurant. (No cheese, mayo, or white bread.)

Quick Meal #5: Belly Fat Free Vanilla Cake Batter Smoothie

Add a scoop of Belly Fat Free Vanilla Cake Batter Smoothie mix and 8 ounces of cold water into a blender. Add a few ice cubes and blend at high speed for 30 seconds. Alternatively, you can use a "shaker bottle" to mix up a delicious Smoothie without the mess or hassle of a blender.

For more recipes, please flip to the end of this chapter (page 177) or visit the forums at BellyFatFree.com.

So there you have it, the complete Belly Fat Free Eating Plan. It's simple, convenient, and very effective. Now it's time for…

BFF Cup Method Summary

1. Eat five mini-meals spaced three hours apart each day.

2. When shopping (and eating), omit foods that contain high fructose corn syrup, stripped carbohydrates, artificial sweeteners, hydrogenated oils and trans fats, excess caffeine, MSG, alcoholic beverages, excess salt, and high amounts of saturated fat—especially if these ingredients are among the first five listed on the label. Also, unless you're eating a food for its good fat content, choose foods that have 25 percent or less of their calories from fat (see page 159 for instructions on how to determine fat calorie content).

3. Choose foods from the Recommended BFF Foods section (beginning on page 154). Have a half-cup protein and one cup of an energy carb for three of your daily meals. For the other two meals, have a half-cup protein and one cup of color carbs. If you weigh 201 pounds or more, see page 163 for portion adjustments. (You can replace one, two, or three meals a day with a Belly Fat Free Smoothie or Belly Fat Free Bar.)

4. Add two tablespoons of healthy oil to your food each day, or eat the recommended foods that are good sources of healthy fat.

5. Drink at least one 12-ounce glass of water before your meal and another during your meal. Sip on water throughout the day, especially when you exercise.

6. If you choose, have three splurge meals during the first week of the program. After that have two splurge meals per week. (If desired—splurge meals are an optional part of the program.)

7. Remember—love the food you eat or you won't stay on the program for long!

BFF Assignment #8 ❏
Start Using Your BFF Eating Tracker

I can't stress how crucial it is to plan and track the foods you're eating in this program by using the BFF Eating Tracker on page 176 (or you can use the online version at BellyFatFree.com). This chart will both keep you accountable and provide a written record of your progress. Be sure to write down *everything* you plan to eat and whether or not you meet your goals. Remember, if you fail to plan you're planning to fail.

Tips for Using the BFF Eating Tracker

❏ Fill in the date, your goal weight, and how many days to your deadline date.

❏ Each night, plan out what you will eat the following day, making sure to include the appropriate amounts of protein, energy carb, and color carb sources for each meal. (Be sure to have all these foods on hand.)

❏ When you meet your goals for each meal, put a check mark in the Met Goal box.

❏ Include notes at the bottom of the sheet about what you did well and what you'll improve on tomorrow.

❏ Take pride in the fact that you're taking action and improving your health and body!

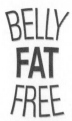

BFF Eating Tracker™

Meal / Time		Source	Met Goal
Mini-Meal One	Protein		☐
	Carb		☐
	Water (oz.)		☐
: AM PM	Supplements		☐
Mini-Meal Two	Protein		☐
	Carb		☐
	Water (oz.)		☐
: AM PM	Supplements		☐
Mini-Meal Three	Protein		☐
	Carb		☐
	Water (oz.)		☐
: AM PM	Supplements		☐
Mini-Meal Four	Protein		☐
	Carb		☐
	Water (oz.)		☐
: AM PM	Supplements		☐
Mini-Meal Five	Protein		☐
	Carb		☐
	Water (oz.)		☐
: AM PM	Supplements		☐

What did I do well today? _____

What will I do even better tomorrow? _____

Belly Fat Free Recipes

The following recipes really are just the tip of the iceberg in terms of all the delicious and healthy options you have on the Belly Fat Free Program. Hundreds of delicious, family-friendly recipes are available in our new cookbook, at BellyFatFree.com/Cookbook. But, for now, here are a few tasty treats to get you started!

Protein Recipes

"Fried" Chicken Tenders

Kids love this recipe, which offers up all the crunch of fried chicken minus the fat. Try dipping the chicken tenders in organic ranch-style dressing for even more flavor.

Ingredients
   1 pound chicken tenderloins
   2 cups plain low-fat yogurt
   ½ teaspoon salt
   ¼ teaspoon pepper
   ½ teaspoon paprika
   2 cups panko bread crumbs or corn flake crumbs

Directions

1. Preheat the oven to 350° F.

2. In a pie plate or shallow dish, mix the seasonings into the yogurt.

3. Put the bread crumbs in another shallow dish. Dip each chicken tender in yogurt, let the excess drip off, and gently roll the tenderloin in crumbs.

4. Bake the chicken tenders on a cookie sheet lined with foil for 15 to 18 minutes. The chicken will be done when the juices run clear.

Baked Marinated Salmon

Salmon is one of the healthiest fish you can eat because it's rich in omega-3 fats. Here's a healthy and delicious way to enjoy it.

Ingredients

Salmon fillets (as many as you'd like)
Roasted sesame seeds (for garnish)
Drizzle of toasted sesame oil (optional)
For the marinade:
½ cup sake
¼ cup tamari sauce (a low-sodium version is preferable)
1 teaspoon fresh grated ginger (sold in jars in produce sections)
1 teaspoon fresh minced garlic

Directions

1. Preheat the oven to 350° F.

2. Combine the marinade ingredients in a small baking pan or heat-safe glass casserole dish.

3. Rinse the salmon fillets and remove any large bones.

4. Place the fillets in the baking dish and marinate them in the refrigerator for an hour. Turn the fish over or spoon marinade over the top of the fillets occasionally so both sides taste good!

5. Bake the fish in the marinade for approximately 8 minutes, then turn the fillets over and bake them for an additional 7 minutes or so (depending on thickness of the fillets).

6. Garnish the fillets with sesame seeds to serve.

Color Carb Recipes

Colorful Steamed Vegetables

Alright, alright. "Steamed" is a misnomer here because we're using a microwave as opposed to actual steam, but the results are very similar and a microwave is faster and easier to use!

Ingredients

Head of broccoli, cut into florets
6 large zucchini, cut to desired thickness
4 large yellow squash, cut diagonally into ¾-inch-wide slices
1 red bell pepper, cut into ½-inch-wide strips
2 medium carrots, peeled and shredded
2 tablespoons fat-free chicken broth (no MSG)
1 tablespoon low-fat parmesan cheese
Salt to taste

Directions

1. Place the vegetables in a large microwaveable covered dish.

2. Pour the chicken broth over the vegetables.

3. Microwave the covered dish on high power until the veggies are tender but not soft (about 8 minutes).

4. Remove the dish from the microwave and, leaving it covered, let it cool for 2 minutes.

5. Season the veggies with parmesan cheese and salt.

Serves six.

Join our free BFF online community at www.BellyFatFree.com

Garlic Tomatoes

This side dish is best with fresh summer tomatoes, but you can make it all year long.

Ingredients

    7 large Roma tomatoes (about 1 ½ pounds), cut in half lengthwise and then cut into ½-inch slices

    2 green onions, minced

    2 large cloves of garlic, peeled and pushed through a garlic press or finely minced

    2 tablespoons red wine vinegar

    2 teaspoons balsamic vinegar

    Salt and pepper

Directions

1. Place the tomatoes in a medium bowl and sprinkle them with garlic and green onions. Mix with a flexible spatula.

2. Drizzle the red wine and balsamic vinegars over the tomatoes and mix with a flexible spatula.

3. Season with salt and pepper to taste.

4. Refrigerate for 30 minutes to allow the flavors to develop.

Serves six.

Creamy Cauliflower Soup

This delicious soup has a delightfully creamy texture and a delicate flavor you won't be able to resist. Even if you think you don't like vegetables, give this recipe a try—it just might change your mind. Oh, and this dish is easy to make to boot!

Ingredients

    1 head cauliflower, cut into 2-inch pieces
    1 large yellow onion, diced
    1 white potato, cut into 1-inch pieces
    4 cups fat-free chicken broth (no MSG)
    3 teaspoons olive oil
    ½ cup low-fat milk (no more than 1%)
    ½ cup (about 4 ounces) shredded fat-free cheddar cheese
    Pinch cayenne pepper
    Salt and pepper

Directions

1. Heat the olive oil in a large pot over medium-high heat until it's simmering (but not smoking).

2. Place the cauliflower, onions, and potato in the pot. Season them with salt and pepper to taste.

3. Cook and stir the vegetables until they are just starting to brown, about 8 minutes.

4. Add chicken stock and bring it to a boil. Reduce the heat to low and simmer until the vegetables are very tender and you can easily push a fork through them, about 30 minutes.

5. Transfer the contents of the pot to a blender. Add the low-fat milk, then blend until smooth.

6. Pour the contents of the blender back into the pot. Stir in the cheese and cayenne pepper. Cook and stir over medium-high heat until the cheese has completely melted.

7. Season with salt and pepper to taste.

30-Second Salad

Enjoy your salad with the simplest and freshest of dressings (not to mention the least expensive!). If you prefer vinegar to lemon juice, by all means, substitute.

Ingredients
Bag of romaine lettuce, chopped
1 lemon
2 teaspoons extra-virgin olive oil
Salt and pepper to taste
Optional: tomatoes, sugar snap peas, broccoli, etc.

Directions

1. Put the lettuce in a bowl.

2. Squeeze a whole lemon over the lettuce.

3. Drizzle with olive oil.

4. Season and add other veggies if you choose.

5. Toss!

Energy Carb Recipes

Spanish Rice

If you're not a big fan of plain brown rice, this is a great way to liven it up…not too spicy but with a nice, zesty tomato flavor.

Ingredients
2 teaspoons olive oil
1 ½ cups brown rice
1 small onion, diced
3 cloves garlic, minced
One 15-ounce can diced tomatoes (preferably organic)
2 ⅔ cups fat-free chicken broth (no MSG)
½ teaspoon cumin
½ teaspoon salt

Directions

1. Heat the olive oil in a large saucepan over medium-high heat.

2. Cook and stir the onions until they're tender, about 5 minutes.

3. Add garlic, then cook and stir until fragrant, about 30 seconds.

4. Add the rice, tomatoes, chicken broth, and salt.

5. Stir the mixture and bring it to a boil.

6. Reduce the heat to low, cover, and simmer for 20 minutes.

7. Remove the pan from the heat, keeping it covered for 20 minutes.

8. Stir the rice before serving.

Herb-Roasted Potatoes

Here's a satisfying goodie! Feel free to play with the herbs in this recipe to customize it to your liking.

Ingredients

5-6 large potatoes, peeled and cut into cubes
2 tablespoons extra-virgin olive oil
2 teaspoons salt
½ teaspoon dried oregano
½ teaspoon dried rosemary
½ teaspoon dried thyme
½ teaspoon onion powder

Directions

1. Preheat the oven to 475° F.

2. In a large bowl, toss the potatoes with olive oil.

3. Sprinkle the potatoes with the spice mixture and toss.

4. Place the potatoes in a single layer on a cookie sheet or roasting pan.

5. Roast for 20 to 30 minutes, turning occasionally.

Baked Sweet Potato "Fries"

If the only way you're used to eating sweet potatoes is in a Thanksgiving casserole, you're missing out on a very nutritious vegetable. Packed with beta carotene, sweet potatoes have a great flavor that can accompany a variety of dishes.

Ingredients
½ teaspoon ground cumin
½ teaspoon salt
¼ teaspoon cayenne pepper
1 tablespoon olive oil
2 large sweet potatoes

Directions

1. In a small bowl, combine the cumin, salt, and pepper. Set the bowl aside.

2. Preheat the oven to 400° F.

3. Peel the potatoes, cut each in half lengthwise, and cut each half into 6 wedges. In a large bowl, combine the cut potatoes, oil, and spice mixture. Toss until the potatoes are evenly coated.

4. On a baking sheet, arrange the potatoes in a single layer and place them on the middle shelf of the oven. Bake until the edges are crisp and the potatoes are cooked through, about 30 minutes. Serve immediately.

Combo Meals: Protein and Carb Recipes

My Favorite Lasagna

This lasagna is one of my personal favorites. Using an all-natural pre-made sauce saves time, and nobody knows the difference!

Ingredients

- 1 8-ounce box of whole wheat lasagna noodles
- 1 10-ounce jar of marinara sauce (choose an all-natural sauce like Barilla, Bertolli, or Newman's Own)
- 1 pound lean ground beef or ground white turkey breast (96% lean)
- 1 24-ounce carton low-fat cottage cheese (1% or less)
- 1 ½ cup mozzarella (2%), shredded

Directions

1. Preheat the oven to 350° F.

2. Begin boiling the water for the lasagna noodles. When it's ready, cook the noodles per the package directions. While you're doing that, brown the ground beef until it's completely cooked. Break it up into small pieces and season them lightly with salt and pepper.

3. Combine the browned beef and marinara sauce in a medium bowl.

4. Once the noodles are cooked and drained, in a lightly greased 9 x 13 casserole dish, begin your layers: put a very light coating of the marinara-beef mixture on the bottom; then place one layer of noodles over that; followed by a layer of sauce; then cottage cheese; and, finally, mozzarella cheese. Repeat these layers, making sure the top layer is cheese.

5. Bake for about one hour (depends on your oven).

Sloppy Joes

Kids of all ages love this quick and tasty version of a family favorite.

Ingredients

    1 large onion, diced

    3 pounds 96% lean ground beef or ground white turkey breast

    8 whole wheat buns (low-fat)

    1 29-ounce can tomato sauce

    1 tablespoon cider vinegar

    1 tablespoon brown sugar (use stevia, truvia™, or Sun
        Crystals™ instead to cut down on sugar even more)

    1 tablespoon paprika

    2 tablespoons Worcestershire sauce

    2 tablespoons modified food starch, mixed with enough water to
        form a slurry

    Salt and pepper

Directions

1. Cook and stir the ground beef and onions in a large heavy skillet until brown, about 10 minutes; drain.

2. Season with salt and pepper to taste.

3. Add tomato sauce, vinegar, brown sugar, Worcestershire, and paprika.

4. Cook and stir over medium heat until the liquid is reduced, about 10 minutes.

5. Add 1 teaspoon starch; cook and stir to thicken. Repeat as required to thicken.

6. Serve on whole wheat buns or toasted whole wheat bread.

Serves eight.

          Belly Fat Free

Turkey Chili

Ground turkey tends to be dry and bland by itself, but this recipe overcomes both of those problems quite handily. Comparable in flavor and texture to a traditional beef chili, this dish is a real crowd pleaser. If you prefer a five-alarm chili just add extra cayenne or chili pepper flakes. This can be served with diced onions and shredded non-fat cheddar cheese.

Ingredients

1 ½ pounds ground white turkey meat
1 onion, diced
2 stalks celery, diced
2 carrots, diced
4 garlic cloves, peeled and minced
1 tablespoon olive oil
1 14 ½-ounce can kidney beans, drained
1 14 ½-ounce can black beans, drained
1 14 ½-ounce can pinto beans, drained
1 29-ounce can diced tomatoes
1 29-ounce can tomato sauce
2 tablespoons cumin
1 tablespoon chili powder
Salt to taste
Black pepper, cayenne, or chili pepper flakes to taste

Directions

1. Cook and stir the onion, celery, and carrots in olive oil over medium-high heat until softened, about 6 minutes.

2. Add the ground turkey and garlic. Cook the turkey until it's just done, taking care not to overcook.

3. Add the remaining ingredients and simmer for 20 to 40 minutes, stirring occasionally.

Serves six.

Beef Stroganoff

This is a delicious and healthy version of the classic Russian dish. The creamy sauce combines the mild sweetness of cooked onions with a hearty beef flavor to create a very satisfying meal.

Ingredients

 1 pound top sirloin steak, thinly sliced and well trimmed of fat
 1 large yellow onion, diced
 8 ounces mushrooms, sliced
 ¾ cup beef broth (low-fat)
 4 teaspoons olive oil (2 teaspoons + 2 teaspoons)
 1 ½ cups sour cream (fat-free)
 2 teaspoons corn starch mixed with enough water to
   make a slurry
 1 pound whole wheat or reduced-carb rotini (spiral-shaped)
   pasta
 Salt and pepper

Directions

1. Heat 2 teaspoons olive oil in a large skillet over medium-low heat.

2. Place the onions and mushrooms in a skillet, season them with salt and pepper to taste, and cook and stir until soft and syrupy, about 20 minutes.

3. Transfer the cooked onions and mushrooms to a small bowl.

4. Fill a large pot halfway with water, cover, and bring it to a boil over high heat.

5. Add pasta to the boiling water, reduce the heat to medium, and cook until tender, about 15 minutes.

6. Heat the remaining 2 teaspoons of olive oil in the same skillet over medium-high heat until simmering (but not smoking).

7. Season the steak with salt and pepper to taste.

8. Cook the steak until it's well browned, about 4 minutes on each side. Transfer the steak to a plate and cover it with foil.

9. Add the beef broth and use a wooden spoon to scrape any brown bits from the bottom of the skillet.

10. Whisk in sour cream and any accumulated beef juices.

11. Remove from heat, whisk in starch, and bring to a boil to thicken the sauce. (Note: You may need more or less starch depending on how thick you want the sauce. If the sauce is too thin, add more starch off-heat and bring it to a boil. If the sauce is too thick, add more beef broth.)

12. Slice the steak into thin bite-sized pieces.

13. Add the steak, onions, and mushrooms into the sauce and mix well.

14. Strain the cooked pasta in a colander.

15. Spoon the stroganoff over the cooked pasta.

Serves four.

One last note: You can make almost any recipe a Belly Fat Free recipe. Adapt recipes from your own kitchen by removing obesity additives, controlling portion sizes, replacing refined grains with whole grains, and substituting healthy lean meats for fatty meats. Be creative!

BFF Success Story
Deborah: Busy Bee Loses the Belly

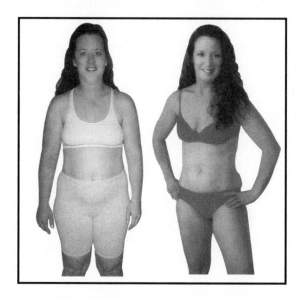

Deborah Wellard is an inspiration for those of us who struggle with balancing wellness with stress and a packed schedule. This 37-year-old mother of two runs a day care center *and* a natural skin care beauty business out of her home. Not only that, but during the 12-week Challenge, Deborah had to deal with her daughter's injury, her niece's death, and her mother's cancer diagnosis. Talk about stress.

In order to take back control of her life, Deborah took a few minutes out of every night to plan out what she would eat the next day; she knew if she didn't do this she would end up eating the wrong foods. And because of her schedule, Deborah had no choice but to exercise at home.

Positive self-talk is a secret that many achievers use, and Deborah is no different. She tells herself, "Others have done this before me, so I know I can do it too!"

Mental strategies such as these helped Deborah get the best of her sugar cravings, and after about two weeks they disappeared altogether. Now she can have a bite of a candy bar for a splurge and say, "Okay, I'm done. I don't need to eat the whole candy bar anymore." When Deborah started the Challenge she was using her splurge meals as a crutch, but as time went on she found she didn't need them that often. "Get the tempting foods out of your house," she advises, "and don't let yourself get ravenously hungry. Eating the five mini-meals per day makes this possible."

Deborah set two-week goals for herself, and found it extremely helpful to avoid weighing herself every day, thus averting discouragement. She realized she was embarking on a new way of living, not a temporary quick fix. As full as her days are, Deborah dedicates five minutes of each and every day to prayer and meditation, concentrating on her body makeover success in the process.

Deborah's mental strength, pre-planning, and regular workouts paid off big. **She lost 49 pounds, 40 ½ inches, and dropped four dress sizes. Her body mass index (BMI) went from obese at 32.1 to normal at 24.4.** And she accomplished all of these extraordinary, life-changing goals by focusing on two-week blocks of time. "One day I noticed my stomach stopped squeezing out of my pants. And then after a while I found I could slip on my red bikini. Now it's fun to look at myself in photographs. I feel good!" she laughs.

Deborah is living proof that what you think affects the way you look.

Belly Fat Free

CHAPTER 8

BFF Approved Supplements

It's no secret that your body requires dozens upon dozens of nutrients—proteins, carbohydrates, vitamins, minerals, trace elements, essential fats, and food chemicals (phytonutrients)—to function *optimally* and maintain good health.

However, the cold hard truth is that most of us are not getting what we need for our short- and long-term health. Not by a long shot. Here's why:

✔ We eat overly processed foods and fast foods that have been stripped of their original nutrient content.

✔ We eat foods grown in nutrient-depleted soils. The vegetables, grains, and fruits grown in these fields therefore lose some of their healthful properties.

✔ Many important nutrients are destroyed in the course of the cooking process.

✔ We lead stressful lifestyles that increase our bodies' demand for certain nutrients.

Let's look at the statistics again. One out of every eight Americans will get cancer. One out of five will develop heart disease. And another one out of four will get diabetes. Not to mention the fact that other diseases like arthritis and osteoporosis are linked to nutritional deficiencies. When we make unhealthy lifestyle choices we put ourselves at risk for every one of these diseases.

On the bright side, an overwhelming number of research studies performed by top doctors at prestigious universities are showing that we have the power to prevent or promote these terrible and debilitating diseases simply by making careful decisions about the food and nutrients we feed our bodies.

With that in mind, taking certain dietary supplements is a really cost-effective way to promote lifelong health and fitness. Taking quality supplements also saves a lot of time and hassle. After all, the alternative is weighing and measuring literally everything you eat, looking it up in a nutrition almanac or database, recording all the information for dozens of nutrients, and repeating the process over and over again. I think you'll agree that this is easily a full-time job.

Furthermore, you'd be eating all day long and, based on how many empty calories are in the typical American diet these days, you'd be taking in so many extra calories in order to get your daily nutrient requirements that you'd end up gaining weight like crazy.

I could go on and on, citing hundreds of supporting scientific studies until we are both bored silly, but the bottom line is this: You need to supplement your diet with, well…supplements. This is true for everyone, but especially for those of us who have a family history of disease and bad health, who are under a lot of stress (and who isn't?), and certainly for those who are trying to transform their bodies by losing fat and adding muscle.

Please believe me when I tell you that, more likely than not, your body is already in a state of nutrient deficiency. When you start to exercise or begin to exercise more intensely, you dramatically increase your body's demand for a wide variety of nutrients like calcium, essential fats, water, amino acids, potassium, sodium, B vitamins, and antioxidants, just to name a few. If you aren't already properly nourishing your body when this happens, you will make the nutrient deficiency even *worse*, thus accelerating the damage.

Get my drift?

Now, whatever you do, don't use this as an excuse not to exercise. Instead, simply follow the Belly Fat Free Eating Plan (from the previous chapter) and add a few simple dietary supplements to your program to cover all your bases.

It really is as simple as that. There's no need to bang your head against the wall, trying to ensure you're getting all the nutrients you need. That isn't a good use of your time or your mental energy. Following the Belly Fat Free Eating Plan and adding a few of the recommendations below will give you all the protection you need.

Recommended Belly Fat Free Supplements

Now that you realize the importance of nutrients (and, therefore, supplements), I want to explain which supplements you really need. Health food stores stock every supplement under the sun, which is enough to completely overwhelm anyone.

Some supplements are good. Many are so-so. Others are completely worthless. Let's take a look at the eight Belly Fat Free supplements that you may want to include in your transformation program.

Supplement #1:
A Quality Nutrition Shake

Nutrition shakes (sometimes called meal replacement powders or protein shakes) are far and away my first supplement choice for anyone who is interested in losing weight and toning her body. Virtually all the men and women you see in this book used nutrition shakes to get great results.

Nutrition shakes provide a quick and convenient way to get in a few of your five mini-meals each day. They're packed with the nutrients necessary to nourish and transform your body and, best of all, they are extremely economical compared to whole foods that contain the same nutrient content. Furthermore, the good ones taste *great*—just like a cold, thick smoothie or milkshake.

But there *is* one thing I have to say up front. **Make sure to read the label of any nutrition shake before you purchase it.** Unfortunately, many of these creamy delights are packed with the obesity additives I've been warning you about throughout this book—high fructose corn syrup, stripped carbohydrates like maltodextrin, large amounts of sugars, low-quality proteins, and unhealthy fats.

Be sure that whatever nutrition shake you use contains an oat flour like Nutrim that is fiber-rich. This energy carb has a gelling effect that causes you to feel full and satisfied quickly—kind of like after you eat a big bowl of oatmeal. But if the product is good it should taste more like ice cream than oatmeal. With Nutrim you also won't experience a surge in your blood sugar levels (which leads to the release of fat-storing hormones and exhaustion). Finally, because Nutrim is made from whole oats, it's heart healthy and has been scientifically shown to support healthy cholesterol and triglyceride levels.

The second fat-fighting ingredient to look for is a calorie-burning and muscle-building nutrient called whey protein isolate—considered to be one of the highest-quality and most absorbable proteins in the world. This protein takes advantage of the thermic effect of foods that we learned about in Chapter 7. Basically this high-quality protein will boost your metabolism by up to 20 percent immediately after you consume it. And of course, this translates to more calories burned...always a good thing! This seems like a good time to mention that a scientific study published in the *Journal of the American College of Nutrition* recently confirmed, once again, that diets higher in protein can help you lose body fat almost *three times faster.*

Tip: Make sure any nutrition shake you choose to use contains an oat flour (like Nutrim) and whey protein isolate.

I've said it before and it's worth mentioning again: Please understand that I'm not recommending a high-protein, low-carbohydrate eating plan by any stretch of the imagination. I recommend a very balanced plan that contains proper amounts of protein, carbohydrates, and good fats. With that said, make no mistake, protein is a very important part of your transformation process. Not only can protein boost your metabolism, it is also the building block of muscle. The truth of the matter is, if you aren't consuming enough protein, there's no way you'll efficiently lose fat and build attractive muscle tone.

Each and every day I talk with good folks from all over the country who aren't eating enough protein. They come to me asking for help, baffled as to why their metabolism is slow and their muscles are withering away (especially vegetarians). But as soon as we start adding a little protein to each of their daily meals, wondrous things happen. They begin to lose weight, feel better, and add muscle.

Recommended use: Enjoy a thick, creamy nutrition shake one to three times daily. Be sure to add a few ice cubes before blending. Find a brand and flavor that meet the guidelines provided in this chapter. I recommend Belly Fat Free Smoothies for their nutrition, taste, and protein/fiber content. Each smoothie contains both a serving of protein (about 20 grams), a serving of energy carbs, good fats, fiber, and a wide array of vitamins and minerals (for more information, see page 169). These smoothies work perfectly in conjunction with the BFF Eating Plan. To order Belly Fat Free Smoothies, simply visit BellyFatFree.com.

Supplement #2:
Fiber

As I've mentioned, it's important to consume around 30 grams of fiber each day. Doing this alone can give you a flat belly, fast. Why? Because fiber (along with fats and proteins) fights belly fat by slowing down the absorption of sugar in the body, which helps fight belly fat, and it helps to cleanse the belly bulge (waste) that comes from an overloaded digestive system.

Fifty percent of Americans aren't getting enough fiber from their daily diet. After all, the American Heart Association recommends 25 to 30 grams of fiber per day to reduce the risk of heart disease. However, most folks are getting only half of that, which is causing digestive problems and increasing their risk of heart disease, diabetes, and certain cancers.

Why is fiber so important for weight loss? Fiber-rich foods make you feel fuller for longer, and they slow the digestion of food so insulin (a fat-storing hormone) is released into the digestive tract. Plus, eating enough fiber (combined with eight to 10 glasses of water a day) keeps your digestive system running smoothly and can clean out pounds of "internal waste" that make your belly bulge. Forget all of those unhealthy laxatives and cleansing detox pills you see advertised…all you really need is an adequate amount of fiber and water.

If you're unable to get 30 grams of fiber from food sources (which is the goal), I suggest supplementing with a product such as Benefiber®, which you can add to any noncarbonated drink. It dissolves completely and doesn't thicken. You can also add this product to soups, sauces, or hot cereals without changing the taste. I also recommend psyllium husks as a great source of fiber. You can take fiber supplements in capsule or chewable form if you prefer. Just make sure they don't contain sugar and other unhealthy additives.

Sprinkling fiber onto high-carb foods slows digestion, thus preventing a surge in fat-storing hormones. This is one of my top tips for people who have a hard time avoiding sweets—add some fiber to your treats.

> Sprinkling fiber onto high-carb foods slows digestion, thus preventing a surge in fat-storing hormones.

Recommended use: Start off with two teaspoons once a day and work your way up to two teaspoons three times a day to add nine grams of healthy fiber to your diet. Add more fiber as necessary to reach a total intake of 30 grams (also be sure to count the fiber you get from food).

Supplement #3: Probiotics

Your body is supposed to be home to trillions of tiny bacteria. And that's a good thing. These beneficial microorganisms serve important functions within the body, mainly within the digestive tract. They do things like ferment foods that we cannot digest (such as fiber), help with elimination, support the immune system, prevent growth of harmful bacteria, and help the body absorb vitamins and minerals. What becomes a problem is when the toxins we have been consuming, as well as medicines like oral antibiotics, have a detrimental effect on these natural bacteria, also called "flora."

Obviously, when the intestinal environment is compromised, digestive side effects may occur. That's why it is common for people taking antibiotics to experience diarrhea, which a 2004 study from Pierre et Marie Curie University in Paris linked directly to the change in gut flora. When "good bacteria" are killed, "bad bacteria" are more likely to take their place and cause problems. A study I talked about in the section on artificial sweeteners found that eating food with Splenda for three months reduced the gut flora in rats. (Maybe it does this in humans, too?)

I recommend adding probiotics and prebiotics to your diet each day in order to maintain the best intestinal environment and reduce your belly bulge quickly. "Probiotics" are foods that either naturally, or because they have been added, contain quantities of beneficial bacteria. "Prebiotics" are foods that contain fiber, which provide nourishment for all those little bacteria.

I recommend sticking to sources that are as natural as possible. Here are some good probiotic foods to consider, and remember, most brands of yogurt contain excess sugar, HFCS, or artificial sweeteners. Avoid them!

- ✔ Stonyfield Farms Oikos Greek Yogurt (plain). Add a zero or low-calorie natural sweetener like truvia™ or Z-Sweet®. Add a high-fiber fruit like raspberries as a bonus.

✔ Lifeway Organic Kefir (plain). This is a drinkable yogurt. Add a splash of vanilla and cinnamon from your spice rack, plus a handful of your favorite high-fiber berries and natural sweetener, if desired. Blend. This makes a great smoothie!

As an alternative, consider trying one of the new shelf-stable probiotic pills, such as Align (Aligngi.com), or Culturelle (Culturelle.com).

Supplement #4:
Omega-3 Fish Oil

Lost in the shuffle of the low-fat diet craze of the 1980s and 1990s was the fact that certain fats are crucial to good health and essential to proper body function. One of these essential fats is omega-3. This good fat is deemed essential because your body cannot produce it; you *must* get it from foods or supplements. The body needs two kinds of omega-3 fats: DHA (docosahexaenoic acid) and EPA (eicosapentaenoic acid).

The benefits of omega-3 fatty acids include:

✔ Reduced inflammation (inflammation can cause body fat due to its effect on insulin)

✔ Balanced blood sugar levels (which reduce cravings)

✔ Increased energy levels

✔ Elevated mood

✔ Accelerated loss of body fat

✔ Improved skin condition

✔ Decreased cardiovascular risk

✔ Reduced symptoms associated with rheumatoid arthritis

✔ Reduced appetite

Who would have thought that a fat could actually help you lose fat? Well, it's true.

The problem is, the best sources of omega-3 fats are cold-water fish including salmon and shellfish, which aren't common staples in the American diet. However, we can survive without having fish sources of omega-3s every day because the body is able to make some EPA and DHA from a different type of omega-3 acid called ALA (alpha-linolenic acid), which is found in whole grains, greens, and some nuts and seeds. But this option isn't ideal because the body can only convert about 15 percent of ALA into the most desired forms of omega-3s.

With all this in mind, I highly encourage supplementation if you want to get all the fat-burning and health benefits of omega-3 fatty acids. Studies back my opinion that omega-3s are one of the best supplement choices around. As for brands, I recommend the Life Extension Foundation® product called Super Omega 3™ available at Lef.org.

Recommended use: Take one 1,000 mg capsule of omega-3 with a meal three times per day. If you need to lose more than 20 pounds, you may increase your dosage to nine capsules total per day. Take three capsules, three times a day to avoid "fish burps" and stomach upset. Alternatively, you can add a tablespoon of Udo's Choice Oil Blend or Barlean's Omega oils (see page 160) to your daily salad or vegetables. Please consult your doctor before starting any new supplement.

Supplement #5:
A Powerful Multivitamin and Mineral

It's sad but true: Your body cells are constantly decaying and dying every second of every day. Unfortunately, the air you breathe and the foods you eat contain deadly toxins, which create evil free radicals that constantly attack and kill precious cells throughout your body. These attacks can lead to low energy levels and poor health. Not to mention other side effects, such as:

- ✔ Damage to your skin including wrinkles, which can make you look older than your actual age
- ✔ Hair loss and damage
- ✔ Weak and fragile nails
- ✔ Inflammation (which many experts believe is the cause of many major diseases)
- ✔ Lowered sex drive
- ✔ Decreased mood and increased stress

What's more, millions of body cells die each day from "starvation." Cells are starved when you don't consume the nutrients necessary to keep your body healthy and full of vitality. Inadequate nutrient intake can also contribute to a host of health problems, including diabetes, heart disease, high cholesterol, and even obesity.

During a meeting of top nutrition scientists at the University of California, a startling idea was proposed: Americans are fat (and getting fatter) not just because they're eating too much, but because they're eating *too little* of some critical nutrients. You see, there are certain vitamins and minerals that are essential to the health of the human body—nutrients we can *only* get by consuming them. If you sit down to a meal that doesn't give your body the nutrients it needs, as I mentioned before, your brain is likely to get the signal to keep on eating until you consume them. This may be why some people are constantly riddled with hunger—they *never* get all the nutrients their bodies need, even if they eat plenty of fruits and vegetables.

What's more, a team of scientists at the Fred Hutchinson Cancer Research Center analyzed survey data from 15,000 people who were asked about their diets, supplement use, and weight changes over the past decade. They were surprised to discover that people who regularly consumed three common nutrients typically gained less weight over a 10-year period than those who didn't. These nutrients included chromium (which helps to balance blood sugar levels that control hunger), vitamin B6, and vitamin B12 (both involved in the conversion of calories to energy).

> Americans are fat (and getting fatter) not just because they're eating too much, but because they're eating *too little* of some critical nutrients.

Additionally, researchers from the University of Rochester reported that overweight and obese children are more likely than children of a normal weight to have iron deficiencies. (Many overweight women are also low on iron.)

Furthermore, according to written accounts from Amanda Prasad, MD, a longtime expert on zinc at Wayne State University, people who don't get enough zinc in their diets lose muscle tissue. Loss of muscle tissue slows the metabolism and causes weight gain. On the other hand, getting enough zinc may help you increase muscle tone and help you lose weight by boosting your metabolism. Still more studies indicate that overweight men and women tend to be low in nutrients such as choline, inositol, and vanadium, all of which play a key role in body fat regulation.

With all this in mind, you have two options to protect yourself from these nutrient deficiencies and free radical damage.

1. You can get all the vitamins and minerals you need by meticulously consuming large amounts of health foods.

Unfortunately, this is something we Americans aren't very good at because it's very difficult to do in this culture. Besides, as we've already discussed, much of the soils our fruits and vegetables are grown in are depleted of nutrients. Thus, so are the crops they bear.

or…

2. You can take a powerful multivitamin and mineral product. But that's only going to work *if* you choose the right one. Read on…

The Problem with Ordinary Multivitamins

Make no mistake, many vitamin products don't make the mark for a number of reasons.

1. Many companies use cheap and ineffective ingredients in their multivitamins (including minerals that aren't chelated or, more technically, are not bound to an amino acid molecule that allows them to be better absorbed by the body), thereby reducing any potential benefit. And, unless you have a biochemistry degree, it's almost impossible to tell the good from the bad. Many grocery and drug store vitamins fall under this category.

2. Many vitamin tablets are pressure packed, which means they won't dissolve when you swallow them. In fact, they may pass right through you. There are actual documented cases where port-a-potties have been emptied and hundreds of undissolved vitamins were found.

3. Many brands leave vitally important nutrients out altogether. Why? Because they don't think you'll notice. This helps them cut costs and make more money. Don't let them get away with this.

4. Tests conducted by an independent consumer protection agency showed that 50 percent of multivitamin and mineral supplements do not contain the nutrients marked on the label. For example, let's say a vitamin label states that it contains 100 percent of the recommended daily allowance (RDA) for vitamin C. Well, tests showed that many brand-name multivitamins contain as little as 10 percent or *no vitamin C at all*. In addition, many multivitamins tested high for potentially dangerous impurities like lead. (Heard of lead poisoning, anyone?)

Now that you know all of this, it's starting to become clear why many of the vitamins you've taken in the past didn't seem to do much except drain your bank account, huh?

Recommended use: When trying to find a good multivitamin, it's really a jungle out there. My best recommendation is to stay away from cheap vitamins found at grocery store chains and discount centers. Instead, buy from independent supplement retailers (like Vitamin Shoppe or GNC) and be sure to check the labels. I also think the multivitamin by the Life Extension Foundation is a good choice (Lef.org).

Especially for Women

A couple of particularly important nutrients for women are iron and calcium, both of which help guard against osteoporosis and anemia. It's especially important to pay attention to these nutrients during weight loss and when under a lot of stress.

Women should shoot for 18 mg of iron and 1,200 mg of calcium per day. (Men typically need a little less, around

---

10 mg of iron and 800 mg of calcium.) Foods rich in iron include lean red meat, legumes, and dark green leafy vegetables. Good sources of calcium-rich foods include dairy products such as low-fat cottage cheese and low-fat yogurt as well as broccoli.

Calcium helps maintain healthy bones, but did you know it also helps support the heart, nerves, muscles, and may even promote weight loss? For starters, a review of studies by the United States National Institutes of Health found that people who are overweight consume much less calcium than people who maintain a healthy weight.

Numerous studies have also linked the reduction of body fat to a higher intake of calcium, particularly in women. A study conducted at Creighton University analyzed the effects of calcium on overweight women of all ages. The study concluded that increasing calcium intake can significantly reduce obesity by as much as 60 to 80 percent.

Another study conducted by Michael Zemel, Ph.D. (a professor of nutrition and medicine at the University of Tennessee) revealed similar results. Two sets of participants were put on a reduced-calorie diet for 24 weeks. One group ingested three to four servings of dairy products in conjunction with practicing a reduced-calorie diet. The other group followed the same low-calorie diet without the added calcium. The results showed that the group consuming approximately 1,200 mg more of calcium per day lost twice as much body fat as those in the low-calcium group.

Supplement #6:
Conjugated Linoleic Acid (CLA)

Conjugated Linoleic Acid (CLA) is a naturally occurring fatty acid found in trace amounts in foods like cheese, butter, and beef. You need to know, however, that these foods don't contain enough CLA to have a positive fat-loss effect. Fortunately, there is a way to purify and extract CLA into gel capsules that contain the proper amounts to help your body naturally fight fat.

One double-blind study, conducted by Thom Erling, Ph.D., gave one test group a dose of CLA at breakfast, lunch, and dinner, while a second group received a placebo. (A placebo is a replacement pill that looks the same but has no active ingredient in it.) After three months the CLA group enjoyed up to a 20-percent decrease in body fat compared to the placebo group, which experienced little change. According to another study in the *American Journal of Clinical Nutrition*, a group of 180 overweight men and women who used CLA lost 9 percent of their total body fat, *without* changing their eating or activity program. Leading CLA researcher, Michael W. Pariza from the University of Wisconsin-Madison, suggests, "In a general sense, what CLA is doing is keeping little fat cells from getting big...perhaps by blocking certain enzymes that let fat cells swell."

Fat normally enters the fat cell through a "door" controlled by an enzyme that acts as a "key." By acting on this enzyme (or key), CLA may keep the door locked, which, in turn, keeps fat from accumulating in the cells. The less fat present in the cells, the smaller and less mature they become, helping reduce the overall level of fat. The increased breakdown of fat helps fuel and preserve muscle mass, which increases metabolism.

Plus, CLA is very safe because it's a naturally occurring fat. This is why CLA is one of my top weight loss supplement choices.

Join our free BFF online community at www.BellyFatFree.com

But you have to be careful about your CLA sources, as it is very easy for unscrupulous companies to fill their CLA gel caps with ordinary vegetable oil.

Recommended use: Take three 1,000 mg gel caps per day, spread out over at least two doses. As with all supplements, check with your doctor before starting a CLA regimen.

Supplement #7: Green Tea

I'm an advocate of green tea for several reasons. First, it contains much less addictive caffeine than coffee. An eight-ounce cup of green tea has between 30 and 50 mg of caffeine, while the same amount of coffee has 95 mg of caffeine. Even worse, energy drinks, soft drinks, espressos, and lattes often contain double to triple the amount of caffeine compared to green tea.

On a national TV appearance, Dr. Nicholas Perricone sparked a big surge in green tea popularity when he mentioned that one could lose weight just by switching from coffee to green tea. He said, "Coffee has organic acids that raise your blood sugar, raise insulin. Insulin puts a lock on body fat. When you switch over to green tea, you get your caffeine, you're all set, but you will drop your insulin levels and body fat will fall very rapidly. So [you can lose] 10 pounds in six weeks, I will guarantee it."

Another reason I like green tea is because many scientific studies have linked it to increased fat burning, as well as prevention of fat absorption. In fact, a 2005 study showed that a supplement containing EGCG (the powerful antioxidant found in green tea) actually prevented obesity in animals by reducing body fat.

If you dislike the taste of green tea or don't want to take the time to make it, you can still reap the benefits by taking a supplement that contains green tea extract. A 1999 study published in the *American Journal of Clinical Nutrition* found that green tea extract boosted the daytime metabolism of test subjects by 35 to 43 percent! Just make sure it's the "extract" version, which is much more potent.

Recommended use: Either drink three to four cups of green tea or take 300 to 400 mg of standardized green tea extract per day. (Those with medical conditions should check with their physician before use.)

Supplement #8: Cinnamon

A study by the USDA Human Nutrition Research Center found that diabetic individuals who took cinnamon after meals all experienced a reduction in blood sugar levels and total cholesterol. The groups taking the highest doses of cinnamon also had reductions in LDL (bad) cholesterol.

This new research on the benefits of cinnamon is the reason many diet pills are now adding this special spice to their formulas. By naturally lowering blood sugar levels, studies indicate that cinnamon may reduce the amount of insulin your body releases. As a result, you may experience less body fat accumulation. Researchers believe this happens because cinnamon has a type of antioxidant that increases insulin sensitivity and effectively stabilizes blood sugar.

With that in mind, if you're planning to indulge in something sweet, the simple addition of cinnamon may prevent your blood sugar from rising as much as it normally would. Feel free to add cinnamon to any food; the benefits of the spice do not diminish after cooking.

Recommended use: Add ⅓ teaspoon of cinnamon to foods one to three times daily. Diabetics, be sure to consult your physician before use.

And that brings us to the conclusion of my top-rated Belly Fat Free Supplements. In conclusion, if you can't afford supplements you can still get amazing BFF results. Many of my success stories featured throughout this book are shining examples of that.

Tip: If your children won't opt for a healthier breakfast option than sugary breakfast cereals, try adding ⅓ teaspoon of cinnamon to the cereal to slow the sugar's digestion. This will keep the kids full longer while reducing fat storage.

BFF Assignment #9 ☐
Accelerate Your Eating and Activity Efforts

If you're like me, you want maximum results in a minimum amount of time. With that in mind, I encourage you to get your hands on a few of the BFF approved supplements listed in this chapter. To help you with your decision, my recommendations throughout this chapter are in order from first to last. And if finances are tight, the fiber, cinnamon, and multivitamin recommendations are very economical.

The Truth About Diet Pills

At this point some of you may be wondering where diet pills fall on my list of recommended products. Believe me, folks, no matter what the advertisement might lead you to believe, **there just aren't any miracle diet pills or potions that will instantly turn you into a stunning supermodel or lean athlete.** Unfortunately, many of today's diet pills—which, incidentally, bring in billions of dollars in sales each year—don't do what they say they will do. Heck, many don't even contain what's indicated on the label.

With that said, there are certain nutrients that may accelerate your progress when combined with diet and exercise. However, I want to take a few minutes to warn you about the tricks and scams many companies use to try and get your money. Being in the know will allow you to make a more educated decision when thinking about using any diet product.

The 7 Deadly Sins of Diet Pills

Deadly Sin #1:
Products disguised to look like prescription weight loss medications.

Diet pills are *supplements*; they are *not* medications. If they were, you'd have to get a prescription to buy them. Many companies try to make their products look and sound like medications in an attempt to trick you into thinking they are prescription-strength. They figure this way you'll think the pills are more powerful and will pay more for them.

There is currently a pill just like this being advertised on TV and radio. The cost? $150 for the exact same type of cheap, ineffective product you can get at your local grocery store for $9. People think products like these *must* work if they are that expensive and sound like a medicine. They are wrong.

The truth is, companies like these often hire actors to pose as doctors and customers. These actors hold up large pants and say how much weight they lost when they really didn't lose any weight at all. They're ripping us off. If these products were really so amazing, why would the companies have to deceive us by making the products look like medications when they're not?

Deadly Sin #2:
Diet pills that make you feel jittery, anxious, depressed, or hungry.

Products like these can cause stress, which leads to emotional overeating and weight gain. They can also negatively impact your health in the long run. Listen to what your body is trying to tell you.

Deadly Sin #3:
Questionable product endorsements.

We talked about this in Chapter 5, and the same rule of thumb applies here: If you wouldn't trust a celebrity to babysit your child, don't trust her advice about a product. Celebrities and doctors are for hire. And, guess what? You're paying their salaries when you purchase the products they're pushing.

Deadly Sin #4:
Diet pills that make outrageous claims.

It's true that the best diet pills are backed by science. However, *no* diet product can help you lose 30 pounds in 30 days. Nonsense. If you're following a quality eating and exercise program and taking scientifically backed weight loss nutrients to speed up the results, you can expect to lose anywhere from eight to 12 pounds per month, depending on how much you have to lose, your age, body chemistry, commitment to the program, and a variety of other factors.

Deadly Sin #5:
Diet products that are not backed by a 100 percent money-back guarantee.

Oh, and also make sure this guarantee lasts long enough that you can actually try the product before it expires (I recommend at least 60 days). This way if the product doesn't work, your bank account doesn't take the hit. After all, if a company isn't confident in their product, why should you be? (Always be sure to read the fine print.)

Deadly Sin #6:
Diet pills that contain token amounts of everything but effective amounts of nothing.

Some diet pills may contain trace amounts of scientifically backed ingredients, but this is only a technicality because they cut corners and only put tiny amounts of these ingredients in the pills—not enough to have a positive effect. This is akin to trying to make a loaf of bread with only a tablespoon of flour.

Look for products that list the amounts of every ingredient on the labels instead of hiding the ingredients in proprietary blends. Then search online to make sure the amounts listed in the products match those recommended by studies.

Deadly Sin #7:
Products that are not tested by independent, third-party laboratories.

This is the *only way* to ensure they contain what their labels say. Here's something you may not know: The Food and Drug

Administration (FDA) does not test supplements to verify the validity of their labels. The scope of this watchdog organization is limited to foods and drugs, which does *not* include dietary supplements.

So who *does* make sure that diet pills contain what their labels say and don't contain any of the bad stuff? Well, it's up to the manufacturing companies to monitor their own products. But most don't. So in all reality, some shameless companies fill their pills with worthless ingredients and charge you 20, 30, 40, or 50 (or more) bucks a bottle for it. Can you believe it? Some companies are cutting corners and padding their wallets by cheating their customers out of the products they're paying for. It's a scam, plain and simple.

Final Thoughts

If you're interested in learning more about what supplements are good and bad, be sure to visit BellyFatFree.com and sign up for my weekly e-mail newsletter. Now that you're armed with all of this knowledge, the tips you're about to learn in the tried and true BFF Transformation Program will really pay off!

BFF Success Story
Angela: My Kids Don't Even Recognize Me In Old Pictures

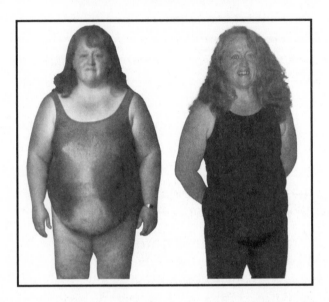

At 37 years old, Angela Silva was sick and tired of her size prohibiting her from getting out and having fun with her family and friends. Even worse, Angela's doctor told her she was headed toward hypertension, diabetes, and even heart disease if she didn't do something about her weight soon.

So Angela decided to participate in the BFF Challenge. She took an active role on the BellyFatFree.com forums, followed the Program, and began to transform her daily routine.

Angela found she had the most success getting in her daily exercise when she did it first thing in the morning. **Soon the pounds and inches began to disappear, and by the end of the first 12 weeks she had lost an amazing 56 pounds and 33 inches, making her the clear winner of that BFF Challenge round.** Her success is amazing, especially considering her hands are full as the mother of seven kids.

But there's more. Angela's success fueled her and, as she explains it, "I had set a goal to lose 124 pounds, and after the first 12 weeks I knew I'd be able to make it all the way."

Sure enough, she kept on going. Today she's lost another 24 pounds, bringing her two-thirds of the way to her ultimate goal. **That's a total of 80 pounds of fat lost.** And knowing Angela, she'll make it all the way to the finish line.

For her, the effort is worth it. Today Angela is uninhibited and enjoys every second she gets to spend being active, having fun with her family. "I have so much more energy, and I just feel happier all the time. Now I go to the park with my kids and I chase them all around the playground. At first when I started doing that, the kids were like, 'Mom, is that you?' My oldest son keeps finding old pictures of me. There weren't many, because I would avoid being in pictures, but when he does find one, he'll say, 'Mom, that doesn't look like you at all!'"

Belly Fat Free

CHAPTER *9*

The BFF Transformation Program

Now before we kick off this chapter, I've got to address an important point. I can already hear the moans and groans coming from some of my readers who really DISLIKE any form of *exercise*. I can hear the excuses piling up already, but remember … excuses are, well … just that, excuses.

Now the "good" news for some of you is that many of my successful students from the past have lost the belly fat without doing exercise. They simply reduced the amount of addicting and fattening obesity additives they were eating and the results soon followed. But if you're like me and you want even *faster* results, read on. I want to share with you my strategies for sculpting and tightening your body in record time.

Moving forward, have you ever wondered how virtually all models and A-list Hollywood actors achieve those incredible celebrity slim, amazingly toned bodies? The answer is **resistance exercise.**

Both resistance (weight lifting) and aerobic exercise (cardio) have tremendous physical and emotional benefits and, as you'll see, the Belly Fat Free Program includes both. But in my opinion, resistance training is the *single* best form of exercise for people who want to reduce their body fat and build calorie-burning muscle fast.

Through resistance training, you can not only sculpt your body quickly but also increase your metabolism. In fact, by adding just five pounds of attractive muscle to your body, you can burn approximately 250 calories a day every day without upping your cardio exercise. (Each pound of muscle you add burns about 50 calories per day.)

Not only will you look better, but studies confirm that resistance training strengthens the heart, increases bone density (which protects against osteoporosis), lowers cholesterol, and even improves mood, which I'm sure we could all use every now and then.

On top of all of that, resistance training doesn't require hours on an exercise bike or in aerobics class. The intensity of resistance training helps you change your body much faster than aerobics alone. In fact, if you do resistance training correctly, you get an aerobic workout simultaneously.

There are really no two ways about it. If you want to look better, feel better, live longer, and stay healthy, resistance training is the key. And ladies, if you're worried that lifting weights will turn you into some sort of inflexible she-man with huge muscles popping out everywhere, don't be. Women on this program create beautiful, shapely bodies like the celebrities you see on TV and in the magazines. I wouldn't have it any other way. (Guys, with this same program you can build a fit, strong, and athletic body. After all, you have the male hormones that allow this to happen.) Now…let's dive into this tried and true program so you can start sculpting a new body.

The BFF Resistance Routine

I want to begin by making one thing crystal clear: **you do not need a membership to a fitness club or recreation center to do**

this workout. Many people perform this program—with amazing results—using basic dumbbells in the comfort and privacy of their own homes, by setting up a simple Belly Fat Free Home Fitness Center. *You don't need fancy equipment.*

I'm certainly not trying to knock gym memberships. If you already belong to a place you enjoy, then by all means use it. I go to a gym occasionally myself, and this program is just as easy to do in a facility as it is at home. If you go to a club, access to exercise machines can be a lot of fun and can add some variety to your workout program.

But I'm going to assume that most of you will be doing this routine at home or at the office (whenever you can steal a few minutes), so let's start with a quick equipment list. Just visit a local used sporting goods store or visit an online source like Craigslist.com or eBay.com to find all the like-new used equipment you'll need.

Equipment Essentials

❏ **Dumbbells:** Sets of 5, 10, 15, and 20 pounds (for women); sets of 10, 20, 30, and 40 pounds (for men). (Both men and women can add more weight as they grow stronger.)

❏ **Workout gloves:** A comfortable pair of workout gloves will protect your hands and help avoid calluses.

❏ **An exercise bench or exercise ball:** You can choose between one of these two options. A quick Google search should turn up a bench for about $75 and a ball for around $20.

The BFF Transformation Program   221

A lot of people ask me if dumbbells (free weights) or machines are a better resistance training option. My general answer is dumbbells. Resistance training with dumbbells allows for the greatest range of motion and can help better your coordination and balance while strengthening muscles that help stabilize joints.

That's it. Pretty simple, huh? If you choose to order online, just grab weighted objects you already have lying around the house and get moving while you're waiting for the equipment to arrive. Or use your own body weight to begin. I want you to start right away. *Don't wait.*

Can You Spare Five Minutes in Front of the TV?

I don't have hours a day to devote to exercise, and I know you don't either. That's why (at least for those of you who haven't exercised in a while) all I'm asking for is five minutes three times a week for the first week. That's it. Feel free to follow this program during the commercial breaks of your favorite TV program if you wish.

Soon we'll work up to 30 minutes three times a week for the resistance training part of this program. However, in the meantime I just want to get you started in the right direction and build some momentum. This may not sound like a lot of time, but our focus is on quality, not quantity. It's about making the most of the time you have to move your body.

If you're new to resistance training and aren't familiar with these exercises, be sure to pay special attention to the step-by-step photos and instructions provided in this chapter. You can also visit BellyFatFree.com to watch video clips of these exercises. If you need further instruction, ask an experienced personal trainer to show you how to properly perform each exercise before you begin. You'll easily get the hang of it in no time (I promise!), so please don't get discouraged.

Once you've mastered this routine—and you will very quickly—visit our Web site for more advanced workouts.

Find a Buddy

Making a commitment to working out with a partner (like your spouse, significant other, or a good friend) is one of the best ways to stay motivated and on track. Inevitably, there *will be* days when you just don't feel like making the effort. However, a training partner will hold you accountable to your goals and vice-versa. If you need a workout buddy, be sure to visit BellyFatFree.com and look in the forum section to find one. Transforming your body is truly a great experience to share.

When to Work Out

I feel the best time of day to exercise is in the morning, before the rest of your life gets in the way. What's more, studies show that exercising first thing in the morning on an empty stomach burns up to 300 percent more fat than exercising during the day, after you've eaten.

If you can't swing this, don't worry. It's more important that you exercise when it's most convenient for you *and* that you're consistent with your efforts no matter if it's morning, noon, or

Sample Workout Schedule

Monday	30 minutes of resistance training
Tuesday	30 minutes of fat-burning aerobics
Wednesday	30 minutes of resistance training
Thursday	30 minutes of fat-burning aerobics
Friday	30 minutes of resistance training
Saturday	30 minutes of fat-burning aerobics
Sunday	Off

The BFF Transformation Program

night. But whatever you do, please don't get in the habit of telling yourself you'll exercise later and then never get around to it. Breaking self-promises erodes your confidence and self-respect, which is the *opposite* of what *Belly Fat Free* is all about.

Now before I unveil the specific details of this program, here's a sample timeline you can follow. I picked Monday, Wednesday, and Friday for resistance training and Tuesday, Thursday, and Saturday for aerobics (covered later in this chapter). Keep in mind, *when* you do this program really doesn't matter. What matters is that you follow through and make it part of your life.

Remember, you can easily adapt this workout schedule to fit *your* specific needs. For example, if you can only squeeze in three exercise sessions per week but you have a little more time for each session, perform your BFF Fat-Burning Routine™ (discussed later in this chapter) *after* your Resistance Routine. Your program would then look like this:

Sample Alternate Workout Schedule

Monday	30 minutes of resistance training 30 minutes of fat-burning aerobics
Tuesday	Off
Wednesday	30 minutes of resistance training 30 minutes of fat-burning aerobics
Thursday	Off
Friday	30 minutes of resistance training 30 minutes of fat-burning aerobics
Saturday	Off
Sunday	Off

There are many ways to structure your activity program. Most important is that you perform three sessions of resistance training and three sessions of fat-burning aerobic exercise each week, no matter how you arrange it.

Some of my clients are so busy they split up their 30-minute resistance routine into three 10-minute sessions. One in the morning, one at noon, and the last at home in front of the TV. You *can* find the time; you just have to make it a priority and always keep your powerful reason to change at the top of your mind.

Before You Begin

Keep the following tips in mind to ensure you maximize the results of your Belly Fat Free Transformation Program.

1. Consult your doctor for a physical examination before beginning this or any other fitness program.

2. This resistance training routine is designed as a circuit program, which simply means that you *move as quickly as possible from one exercise to the next*. Rest only long enough to get set up for the next movement. This simultaneously burns more calories and strengthens your heart.

3. Try to increase the amount of weight used each week, but don't sacrifice your form in the process. If you can't maintain proper form when increasing the weight, it's too heavy. But don't go too light either. The more you challenge yourself, the faster you'll see results.

4. Keep each movement slow and controlled. Both the positive (or lifting) and negative (or lowering) parts of each exercise should take two seconds (one-thousand-one, one-thousand-two). Also, pause for one second at the top. So again: you'll lift for two counts, hold for one, lower for two.

5. Don't hold your breath during the exercises. Your muscles need the oxygen now more than ever, so *breathe deeply*.

6. If you're new to fitness, one circuit may be enough at the beginning. But add another circuit as soon as you can until you reach three circuits.

7. Be sure to warm up for a few minutes before your resistance workout—something simple like marching in place or walking up and down stairs will do. Then stretch out for five minutes afterward.

8. Strive for at least eight hours of sleep each night to ensure recuperation.

9. Nourish your body with healthful foods by following the BFF Eating Plan from Chapter 7.

10. Absolutely, positively *track your progress* using the BFF Transformation Tracker progress report found at the end of this section (page 246).

Gym Jargon Revealed

Let's talk about a few terms. Lifting a weight up and lowering it down once is called a *repetition*. The Belly Fat Free Resistance Routine includes 10 repetitions for each exercise.

You'll need to select a weight for each exercise that you can repeat no more than ten times. If you're still cranking at 12 or 15 repetitions, it's time to increase your weight. After all, the amount of weight you use has to be heavy enough to get those muscle cells' attention and cause them to adapt and grow. Each group of repetitions is called a *set*.

So here's your goal:

1. Complete one set of 10 repetitions for each exercise. All the sets of all exercises together equal one *circuit*. Remember, to build confidence during the first week you can choose to do only five minutes of this routine, three times per week.

2. As soon as you feel comfortable, repeat the whole sequence over again, completing a second circuit and then a third.

Intensity Booster

To really boost your Belly Fat Free Resistance Routine results, try a secret intensity booster that I affectionately call the BFF Peak Intensity Technique™. Here's how it works: For every set of each exercise, once you've successfully blitzed your muscles for a tough 10 reps, call on your inner strength for one more half-rep and push the weight to the lifting phase midpoint (or halfway point) of whatever exercise you're performing and hold that position for five seconds.

Sounds simple enough, but if you've truly challenged yourself for the first 10 reps like you should have, that eleventh "static rep" will be super tough. It's intense but, believe me, it works to build your body fast. And fast results are the goal.

Begin by performing one to two circuits of all the exercises. However, if you're participating in the Belly Fat Free Challenge (And why not? Fame, fortune, and fulfillment are all at your fingertips—not to mention prizes!), you'll definitely want to bump up the intensity by adding a third circuit as soon as you can. Remember, you started this program because you were tired of the old you. The more you put into it, the better the results you'll get.

Not sure how much weight to use? Just start with a five-pound dumbbell and see what it feels like. You can go up from there. You'll most likely use more weight for compound movements (exercises like a chest press that involve many muscle groups) than you will for simple movements (exercises like a bicep curl that isolate a muscle group).

For example, the One-Arm Row back exercise (page 230) is a complex movement because it uses muscles in your back, shoulders, and arms; the Triceps Kickback exercise (page 232) is a simple movement involving mainly your triceps (located on the back of your upper arms). Believe me, you'll be able to use a lot more weight for Rows than you will for Kickbacks.

Okay…let's get started!

The Belly Fat Free 10

These 10 exercises will be a wake-up call for your muscles. Keep each movement slow and controlled and repeat each one 10 times (10 repetitions). Then put the pedal to the metal, crank up the intensity, and hold that eleventh static rep at its midpoint during the BFF Peak Intensity Technique rep.

You can easily do these exercises at home, in front of the TV, whenever you have a few minutes. You can also use an exercise ball instead of a weight bench for any of these exercises.

Exercise #1: Chest Press

Muscles worked: Chest

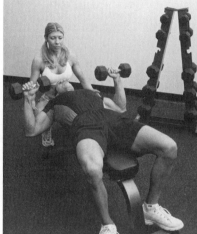

Start

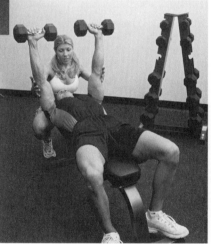

Finish

Instructions: Grip a dumbbell in each hand, with your palms facing forward. Lie back on a flat bench or exercise ball with the dumbbells close to your chest and your feet flat on the floor. As you exhale, push the dumbbells up (palms still facing forward) until the dumbbells touch. Pause for a second and inhale as you slowly lower the dumbbells toward the starting position, stopping when your upper arms are slightly below parallel with the floor.

Join our free BFF online community at www.BellyFatFree.com

Exercise #2: One-Arm Rows

Muscles worked: Upper and middle back

Start

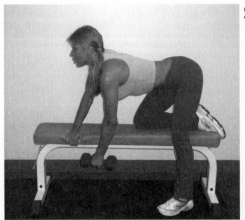

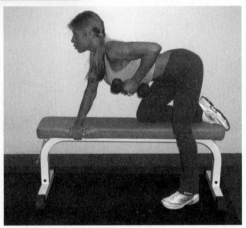

Finish

Instructions: Begin with your right hand and knee on a flat bench, and your left foot on the floor with the knee slightly bent. While gripping the dumbbell in your left hand, keep your back flat and your head in a neutral position. Pull the dumbbell up toward the side of your waist, keeping your elbow pointed to the ceiling and pulling your shoulder blade toward the center of your back. Once complete, repeat with the other arm.

Exercise #3: Seated Overhead Press

Muscles worked: Shoulders

Start

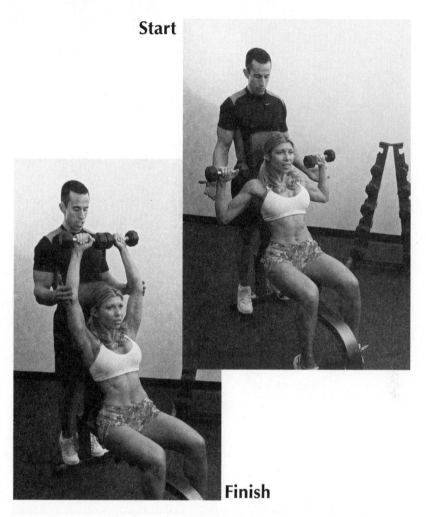

Finish

Instructions: Sit on a bench or an exercise ball, abs tight, a dumbbell in each hand, elbows at shoulder level, and bent to 90 degrees. Your palms should face forward as you slowly press the dumbbells up and together. Keep just a slight bend in your elbows at the top, then slowly lower your arms until your upper arms are slightly below parallel to the floor.

Exercise #4: Triceps Kickbacks

Muscles worked: Triceps (backs of upper arms)

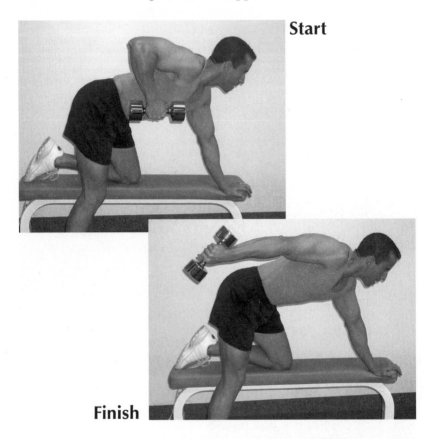

Start

Finish

Instructions: Place your right knee and your right hand on a sturdy chair or bench for support. Pick up a dumbbell in your left hand, palm facing in. Your left foot should stay flat on the floor. Hold your left arm close to your rib cage, then extend the dumbbell back and away until your arm is parallel with the floor. Tighten your triceps at the top, then slowly lower your arm to the starting position. When complete, repeat on the other side.

Exercise #5: Seated Biceps Curls

Muscles worked: Biceps (fronts of upper arms)

Start

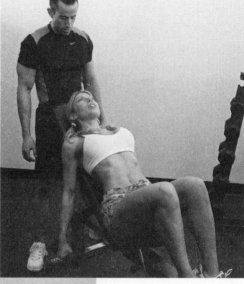

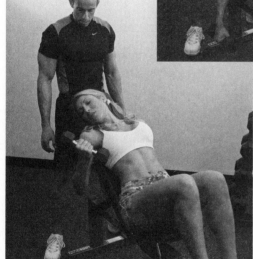

Finish

Instructions: Sit on a bench or an exercise ball and hold one dumb-bell in each hand with your palms facing inward, elbows close to your body. Slowly rotate your palms up as you lift the dumbbells toward your shoulders. Contract your biceps at the top, then slowly lower the dumbbells back to your sides while rotating your palms inward.

Exercise #6: Lunges

Muscles worked: Thighs and glutes

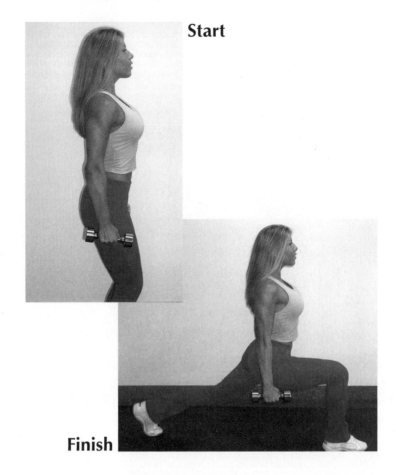

Start

Finish

Instructions: Stand with a dumbbell in each hand, arms at your sides. With your head up and back straight, step back with your left foot, a little wider than a normal step, while lowering your left knee to the ground. Your right knee should also bend as you dip down. Bring the left leg forward and repeat with the right leg. One repetition consists of a pair of lunges (i.e., one on the right and one on the left).

Exercise #7: Squats

Muscles worked: Thighs and butt

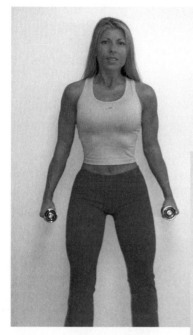

Start

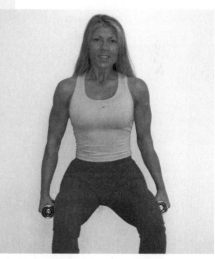

Finish

Instructions: Stand with your feet about hip-width apart, heels pressed down firmly. Hold a dumbbell in each hand and slowly bend your knees, keeping your back straight until you reach a position where your thighs are parallel to the floor, then return to your standing position. Be sure that your knees do not extend forward past your toes (do this by sitting back into the position as if you were sitting into a chair).

*If the exercise is too difficult with dumbbells, try it without them first, then add weight once you get stronger.

The BFF Transformation Program   235

Exercise #8: Standing Heel Raises

Muscles worked: Calves

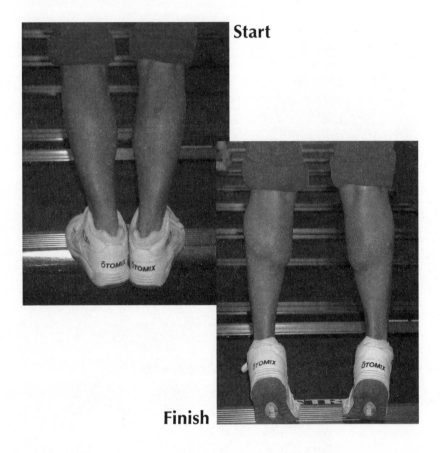

Start

Finish

Instructions: Stand with your feet about hip-width apart on a stair. Move to the edge of the stair so that everything from the balls of your feet up to your toes is supported but your heels are unsupported. Grip a rail or something to keep your balance and slowly push up on your toes. Pause at the top and concentrate on contracting your calf muscles. Then slowly lower your heels down until you feel a comfortable stretch in the back of your calves and ankles.

Exercise #9: Double-Leg Stretch

Muscles worked: Abdominals

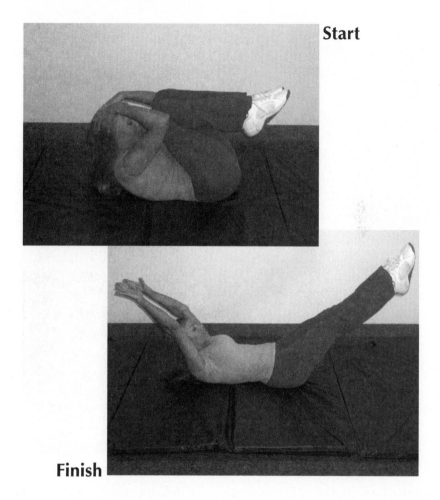

Start

Finish

Instructions: Lie on your back with both knees pulled in toward your chest. Lift your head and neck with your chin tucked. Exhale and feel your navel sink toward your spine. Inhale and reach your arms long behind you at an angle, with your legs in front at about 45 degrees. As you exhale, bring your knees in to your chest and circle your arms around to meet them.

The BFF Transformation Program   237

Exercise #10: The Bicycle

Muscles worked: Abdominals

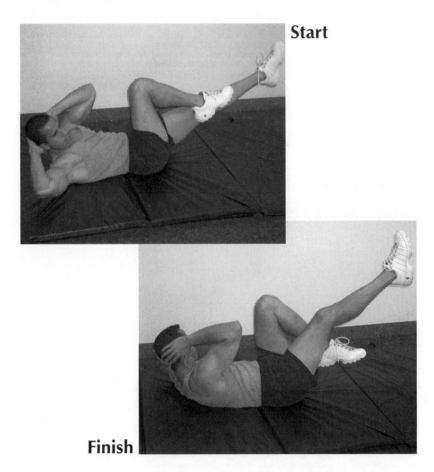

Start

Finish

Instructions: Lie on your back with hands behind your lifted head and knees in toward your chest. Extend your right leg out and up on an angle. Inhale and slowly twist your upper body until your right elbow touches your left knee. Look back toward your left elbow and hold the position as you exhale. Switch to the other side, bringing your left elbow to your right knee, as you extend your left leg. Both sides together count as one repetition.

That's the Belly Fat Free Resistance Routine. It doesn't sound too difficult, now does it? Remember, this workout should take about 30 minutes (three circuits), and you only need to perform it three days a week for excellent results. Also, don't forget to increase the weight used for the exercises as you grow stronger.

And just a reminder—don't forget to use the BFF Transformation Tracker (page 246) to monitor and track your progress throughout the 12-week program. This same chart is also available online at BellyFatFree.com.

The BFF Fat-Burning Routine

The fat-burning (or aerobic exercise) component of the program is very simple and straightforward. No voodoo or crazy exercise contraptions necessary. Here's how it works: Perform 30 minutes of fat-burning aerobic exercise, such as walking, jogging, biking, swimming, kick boxing, or stair stepping, three times a week. The activity type is completely up to you; just be sure you pick a type of aerobic exercise you really enjoy, something that sparks your interest. And don't be afraid to cross train.

For example, I love to hike briskly in the foothills behind my Colorado home in the spring, summer, and fall. But, as much as this activity thrills me, I still want a change every once in a while. So I go for a run with a buddy, play a friendly game of basketball, or ride my exercise bike in the morning while watching educational DVDs or the occasional movie. (I don't like watching regular TV because of all of the commercials for fast food. These commercials really do cause cravings.)

I've worked with many people who enjoy going to dance classes. One of my friends even plays competitive racquetball because he can't stand traditional aerobic exercise. The important thing is to be *active* and get that heart rate up. **The only rule is no excuses.** Thoughts like, "I'll do it later," or "I'll do it tomorrow," or "the weather isn't nice enough" do nothing more than excuse you from having the body you really deserve.

I also use this time in my day to practice my BFF Confidence Booster. For example, if I'm on a bike ride or walk, I'll listen to a recording made to help guide me through this valuable reprogramming technique (see Chapter 3 for a refresher on this). This brings a lot of confidence and happiness to my life, and I do it almost every day. I hope you will too. Believe me, you'll feel so much better once you start. You'll have more energy, your mood will improve, your confidence will jump, health problems will vanish, stress levels will subside, and your fat will shrink. What could be better than all that?

When you consider that the average American is parked in front of the TV for a staggering 30 hours a week (and we wonder why more than 100 million adults and 20 million children are overweight in this country!), what I'm asking for isn't much. Heck, you can even do this routine while watching TV if you want. During these aerobic sessions, you'll be focusing your efforts on burning body fat. But here's the catch…

You Gotta Change Your Pace

Here's the scoop: Researchers have found you can dramatically boost your metabolism, not only during your workout, but also for hours afterwards when you change the pace or intensity of an exercise. It's true.

Whatever you do, do *not* remain at one pace during your entire aerobic session. For example, when I'm on the treadmill I like to start by walking at a moderate pace for a minute, then I work up to a jog for a minute, then I sprint for a minute…and repeat the

240   Belly Fat Free

sequence. It really breaks things up, burns a lot of calories, and the workout is over before I know it. Just remember to go slow, medium, and fast for each minute until your time is up.

Make no mistake, you can burn a lot more calories in 30 minutes of varied-intensity aerobics then an hour of slow-motion movement. Fast results match my overall philosophy when it comes to transforming bodies. I want maximum results in minimum time…and I'm sure you do too. After all, why take a year to transform your body when you can achieve the same results in just 12 weeks or less?

A constant variation in pace and activity type really keeps me motivated. It's also a great way to burn body fat because you're constantly challenging yourself rather than settling into a routine. Your heart will be pumping and you'll practically feel the fat melting off your body with each drop of sweat. Try it for yourself—you'll know what I'm talking about.

Remember, if you're a beginner who hasn't exercised in a while, take it easy for the first few sessions of this program. Maybe you'll only be able to start with five minutes. If so, don't worry! You can build your way up as you go along. Just remember to push yourself so you *really* burn that unattractive body fat.

That's it. By doing this you'll burn all that stored blubber that's been haunting you for years. You'll take back control of your body, and after a few days this activity will become *addicting*. Your body releases all kinds of feel-good hormones when you exercise. At first you won't be in tune with these feelings because your body isn't used to moving intensely. But soon this exercise will become a very uplifting experience. You'll crave aerobic activity, and it will act almost like a jackhammer, blasting away old food cravings and addictions.

What's more, you'll soon find that your stress levels decrease significantly, depression lifts, you'll be happier, and you'll begin to think more clearly. Exercise has been proven to stimulate brain activity; think of your mind lighting up like a Christmas tree. It's an amazing miracle that most of us have taken for granted at some point in our lives…but not anymore!

Consider this: Our bodies were designed to move. But when we don't use our bodies like they were designed, we start to feel badly and our bodies start to look bad. The old maxim "If you don't use it, you'll lose it" really is true. It's a good thing we have the ability to regain what we once lost even after decades of inactivity and abuse. When it comes to exercise, the human body is a truly amazing machine that adapts to the challenges placed before it.

Defining Aerobic Activity

People constantly ask me if gardening, housework, or walking during work can take the place of their BFF Fat-Burning Routine. My response is that these activities are just that—activities. They *do* burn more calories than just sitting, but they aren't intense enough to really help you lose weight and increase your cardio-vascular health (heart health) unless you're performing them at an intense level (around a seven on the intensity scale of one to 10) for 30 minutes.

The point I'm trying to make is this: Please don't try to weasel out of doing this aerobic routine by trying to rationalize that taking that flight of stairs at work or walking half a block to your car makes up for it. Sorry, but it doesn't work that way. I'm bound and determined to help you get great results, so I have to really lay it on the line.

Again, I want to recommend that you try to exercise first thing in the morning before you eat breakfast. After fasting overnight your body's blood sugar levels will be naturally lowered. Therefore, when you start exercising, your body will be forced to dip into your stubborn fat cells to fuel your movement instead of burning the blood sugar from foods you've recently eaten. Again, remember that by doing this one simple trick, you can burn fat up to 300 percent faster than you could if you performed the same exercise later in the day, after you've already eaten. This is an important secret for those looking to exercise less and get better results.

> **Tip:** If you feel nauseated or dizzy while exercising on an empty stomach, try having a non-carbohydrate food (like a few almonds or some low-fat cottage cheese) right after you wake up. This will settle your hunger without dramatically increasing your blood sugar levels. And *always* start your day with a tall glass of water.

So, there you have it—the complete Belly Fat Free Transformation Routine. Once you've mastered it, you'll be well on your way to creating the body you deserve once and for all. **I encourage you to consider each exercise session a victory in your quest to improve your body and your life.** Track your progress using the chart on page 246, or use the online version available at BellyFatFree.com. Celebrate your progress, *have fun with the program,* and make it an empowering experience each and every day.

BFF Assignment #10 ☐
Drop and Give Me Ten

Your next assignment is to get your body moving...right now. I'm serious. One of my "life rules" is to always take action as soon as possible. If I learn something that I think will benefit me, I don't wait to make a move. I write an e-mail, make a call, or do something—*anything*—to capture that magical momentum and get the ball rolling.

So right this instant, I'm asking you to do the same thing. Let's get your heart beating, let's fill your lungs with vitalizing oxygen, let's get your muscles moving. I'm asking for 60 seconds. Are you with me? If so, simply do 10 push-ups—even if you have to do them on your knees to begin. (If you can't do 10, do what you can. You will improve!) Then I want you to either jog in place intensely for 30 seconds or find a staircase to climb for 30 seconds.

That's it. When you're done, give yourself a big pat on the back and be proud. Notice the surge of energy and alertness you feel. Congratulations! You've stepped onto a path that will take you to where you want to go.

Tips for Using the BFF Transformation Tracker

❑ Fill out the date, start time, and finish time each time you perform the BFF Resistance Routine.

❑ Your Goal Reps for each exercise will be eleven (including the eleventh static rep for the BFF Intensity Technique).

❑ Under Weight Used, record the weight of the dumbbells used.

❑ Write down the number of completed movements for each listed exercise in the Reps Done section.

❑ Three extra exercise spaces have been provided so you can add in more exercises if you're feeling ambitious.

❑ Write down the aerobic exercise you plan to do in the BFF Fat-Burning Tracker section (be sure to include the duration as well). If you meet your goal, put a check mark in the Met Goal box. This section includes three blank spaces in case you break your fat-burning work into multiple sessions throughout the day. (Some people like to do three 10-minute activity sessions at morning, noon, and night, respectively.)

❑ Write down any questions and notes about your workout at the bottom of the Tracker.

❑ Pat yourself on the back and give yourself credit for following through and taking action!

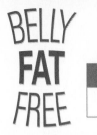

BFF Transformation Tracker™

Date:	Start Time:	Finish Time:

BFF Resistance Routine™	Circuit 1			Circuit 2			Circuit 3		
	Goal Reps	Weight Used	Reps Done	Goal Reps	Weight Used	Reps Done	Goal Reps	Weight Used	Reps Done
Chest Press									
One-Arm Rows									
Seated Overhead Press									
Triceps Kickbacks									
Seated Biceps Curls									
Lunges									
Squats									
Standing Heel Raises									
Double-Leg Stretch									
The Bicycle									

BFF Fat Burning Tracker™	Exercise	Duration	Met Goal
			☐
			☐
Date:			☐

What did I do well today? _____

What will I do even better tomorrow? _____

Notes: _____

Join our free BFF online community at www.BellyFatFree.com

BFF Success Story
Linn: Overcoming Physical Limitations to Win the Challenge

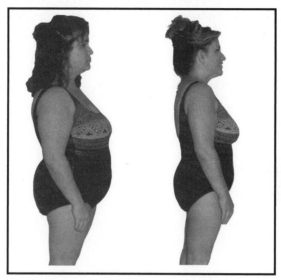

Linn Ash, a 44-year-old licensed massage therapist and mother of two, had several health issues that went hand in hand with her weight problem. Fearful of exercising because of her arthritis, she had chosen a path that involved no exercise, which caused her to gain weight and made other health issues even worse.

Linn read *Belly Fat Free,* and newly determined, she developed an activity plan that she could do even when she was limited by joint pain. She also became a very active member of the BellyFatFree.com forums. Long before she was selected as Round Winner in the BFF Challenge, Linn was coaching, encouraging, and cheering her online friends along.

By the end of her Challenge, Linn lost 40 pounds and 42 ½ inches. She was able to trade in her size 18 jeans for a petite six. Even better, she noticed improvements in her health as well. All of

Join our free BFF online community at www.BellyFatFree.com

her hard work paid off in other ways too; as a Round Winner in the BFF Challenge Linn won thousands in cash and a Caribbean cruise getaway for two.

"I want to be an inspiration for everyone to make the decision to start losing weight today. There really is no reason to continue feeling miserable and fat when BellyFatFree.com provides all the tools you need to become healthier and learn a better way of feeding both your body and your family."

Chapter 10

A New Beginning

I'm proud of you. I really am.

Most people never make it this far. They put their time and effort into seeking out all of this valuable life-enhancing information and then let it sit and gather dust or read it and don't take action. But you're different, my friend. That's why I have a great deal of confidence in your ability to succeed.

Believe me, there's no better time to get going than *right this instant*—not tomorrow, or next week, or next month—but right now. If you wait until everything is perfect in your life, you'll be waiting forever. And I don't want you to delay the pleasure of having a new you. Please don't think you'll be doing this all alone because...

I'm Here to Support and Guide You Every Step of the Way

Remember at the very beginning of this book when I told you I was here to help, that I refuse to let you fail? Well, I was very serious. That's why if you have any questions at all—or even if you just need a little encouragement—I'd enjoy hearing from you. At any time, day or night, please visit BellyFatFree.com and post a message in the forums or journals. I visit frequently, and we have a whole team of folks dedicated to lending a helping hand.

Another way I can keep in touch with you is through my complimentary Belly Fat Free e-mail newsletter (available by signing up at BellyFatFree.com). In each issue you'll receive late-breaking news about new ways to battle the bulge, weight loss breakthroughs, and inspiring updates on our most recent success stories. (Just think, soon you may be one of them!)

You know, I've discovered that many people read this book all the way through and have great intentions to start shaping up the next day. But then life takes over and, before they know it, months have passed and they're still stuck in a body they are miserable with. It's vitally important to take action *right now*. With this in mind, the following final Belly Fat Free Assignment is perhaps the most important of all. Please promise me you'll do it right now?

BFF Assignment #11 ☐
Cross the Finish Line

Go back through this book and be sure to accomplish all the previous BFF Assignments. Completing these tasks really *is* the key to achieving all you want out of life...and more. Everything you need to succeed is right here, in your hands.

Final Thoughts

Most of us weren't taught about the importance of food when we were children. We ate what appealed to us the most, and we grew accustomed (many times addicted) to these foods, so much that natural foods didn't taste good in comparison.

But remember, the human body is a complex machine that requires a wide variety of nutrients to remain healthy. Nutrients like proteins, essential fats, carbohydrates, fiber, water, vitamins, and minerals. Without the proper amount of these nutrients, we develop deficiencies and our bodies don't function properly. Our minds become clouded, we can't handle stress, we get colds, we can't sleep, our bodies ache, and our energy levels plummet.

After a while in this deprived state, the human body *will* break down—diseases like diabetes, cancer, osteoporosis, arthritis, and heart disease set in and our quality of life is shattered. That is, if our lives aren't ended completely.

But we have a choice about what we put into our bodies. Food *really does* make or break us. It can help us be healthy and happy, or it can make us sick and depressed. It can energize us or it can make us lazy. It can make us look attractive and feel confident or force us to look unattractive and feel insecure.

It's our choice. And what we teach the children of this country is also our choice. Know that filling kids up with junk food on a consistent basis isn't a rite of passage or a harmless treat. It's literally a one-way ticket to future sickness, obesity, and despair.

Many health experts agree that allowing children to consistently eat obesity additives is more harmful to their health than letting them smoke cigarettes. It's your choice: a pile of trans fat-laced French fries, a bowl of Sugar Bomb cereal, or a Joe Camel.

They're all slow killers. It bears repeating that obesity has overtaken cigarette smoking as America's number-one preventable disease.

The number of overweight children today has quadrupled since the 1970s, and it keeps getting higher. What's more, 80 percent of all overweight children will go on to be overweight adults. With that in mind, I encourage you to pass along the information you've learned in *Belly Fat Free* to the children in your life. It's not up to the schools to educate America's kids about how to eat… it's up to us.

And finally, I encourage you to clean up your "toxic zone" by replacing any junk food in your house with nutrient-dense "fun food." I call healthy food "fun food" because life is so much more enjoyable when you're healthy, confident, and looking your very best.

Just some food for thought…

I sincerely hope you've gotten a great deal of value and knowledge out of *Belly Fat Free*. I hope you'll share all that you've learned with your friends and family members too so that we can create a united front to shape up America and transform that overweight and depressed Statue of Obesity from the front cover back to a symbol of liberty, hope, and happiness for all.

Please let me know all about the progress you've made as you work through this program. It would really mean a lot to me; I love hearing from people just like you—people who are putting forth the effort to really change and better their lives. You can leave a post for me at my Web site BellyFatFree.com or e-mail me at Support@BellyFatFree.com. Please be sure to include "before" and "after" photos if you have them.

As this book draws to a close, I hope this won't be the end of our relationship but rather the beginning—the first step on the path to your incredible success.

Frequently Asked Questions

Following are some of the more common questions about the Belly Fat Free Program. If you have a question not covered here, please contact a Coach online at BellyFatFree.com.

Q: *Can you tell me more about the BFF Challenge and how I can win cash and prizes just for getting slim?*

A: Here it is in a nutshell: You'll have 12 weeks to follow the Belly Fat Free Program, transforming your body and your life in the process. Then you'll report your results to us at BellyFatFree.com to claim your chance at an amazing prize package. I could go on and on about this incredible transformation challenge, but the simplest way to get all the information you need is to review the complete Rules and Regulations Guide online. Nationwide, men and women of all ages and fitness levels are making incredible life-changing transformations. I'm convinced you can, too. (Note: The Belly Fat Free Challenge is void in some states. Please see the complete Rules and Regulations Guide at BellyFatFree.com/Challenge for details.)

Q: *Eating five times a day seems like a lot. Are you* sure *about that? Wouldn't I achieve more rapid results if I skipped some meals?*

A: No, you wouldn't. It's as simple as that. Even though the concept may seem odd, it really is better to have a meal every three hours...as long as each meal is small. (Sorry, we're not talking about all-you-can-eat buffets.) Revisit Chapter 7 for ideas on how to gauge appropriate food portion sizes and some sample menus.

Skipping meals leaves you feeling drained, hungry, and cranky. Plus it sends your body the message that it should slow your metabolism in order to conserve energy (which means it holds onto fat stores). Frequent healthy meals, on the other hand, have many benefits, such as:

- ✔ Staving off starvation cravings
- ✔ Stabilizing blood sugar so you feel more energetic
- ✔ Keeping your metabolism cranked up so you burn more calories
- ✔ Providing a constant fuel supply to feed that muscle tissue you're creating
- ✔ Keeping fat-producing hormones in check

Trust me on this. Five meals a day is the way to go.

Q: *Do I have to do the exercise portion of the BFF program?*

A: Nope. You can lose weight without doing it, but I have to warn you that it will take longer and your body won't look nearly as good when you're done. I want you to get amazing, fast results, so do some form of activity that you love, okay?

Q: *My schedule is so crazy that I usually end up eating dinner late, like around 9 p.m. Is that okay?*

A: Well, not really, unless you plan to be up and moving around for another three hours after you eat. With all the demands on our time, though, it's easy to understand how eating gets pushed off until later.

But if you eat at 9 p.m. then go to bed an hour later, what happens to that food? Is it burned to fuel your activities? Probably not. Most likely you've got some really happy fat cells just soaking it all in while you're snoozing.

My best advice is to stop eating three hours before bed. If you do need something to munch on or you have to eat right before bed, choose from a quality protein source with a color carb selection. A little low-fat cottage cheese with some sliced grapes or pineapple works great for me.

Q: *My budget is pretty tight, and I don't think I can afford all the supplements discussed in Chapter 8. If I can only afford one, which would you suggest?*

A: That's tough because all the products help bolster your improvements in different ways. But if you can only use one, I think Belly Fat Free Smoothies are hard to beat.

We're talking complete, balanced nutrition in one super-convenient and delicious smoothie. From the special protein blend designed to kick-start your metabolism to a staged-release carbohydrate blend to ensure a smooth energy supply and stable blood-sugar levels (a major bonus for fat loss), Belly Fat Free Smoothies have it all. Top it all off with a balanced serving of 24 vitamins and minerals and you've got a powerful fat-loss support weapon that helps you feed your body consistently throughout the day. They're available at BellyFatFree.com.

Q: *What if I want to add or substitute exercises besides those recommended in this book? Can I do that and, if so, what exercises would you recommend?*

A: You *absolutely* can add or substitute exercises. Once you've mastered the BFF Resistance Routine exercises, the sky's the limit. As a matter of fact, variety is key to your success with any exercise program. Visit BellyFatFree.com for more advanced programs.

Q: *What if I can't complete all the resistance exercises in the beginning?*

A: *That's okay.* Anything you can complete is better than no exercise at all, but also keep in mind that the more quickly you work up your strength to the point where you can do all the exercises, the faster you'll see results.

The most important thing is to make the commitment, get started, and do the best you possibly can. Here are some options for ways to modify the Resistance Routine until you can get through a complete circuit:

✔ Do a reduced number of repetitions, but at least a few reps of each movement.

✔ Use very light weights or no weights at all until you're strong enough to add them.

✔ Try some of the alternative exercises. Everyone is different, and some movements may be easier for you to start with than others.

Q: *What if the BFF Resistance Routine is too easy for me and I want more of a challenge?*

A: Let me start by saying good for you! That means you've exercised seriously in the past, which is great.

One of the things I like so much about the Belly Fat Free Program in general is the flexibility—and the Resistance Routine is an excellent example of that. To make this routine more difficult, you've got several options:

✔ Simply increase the amount of weight you're lifting.

✔ Add another circuit.

✔ Move through the circuit even faster, with less rest between sets.

✔ Add some of the alternate exercises.

✔ As for the Fat-Burning Routine, try a type of exercise you haven't done before or increase the intensity of your effort.

Q: *How come these workouts are so short? My best friend spends hours at the gym and, even at that, she still hardly ever reaches her goals.*

A: What the heck is she doing in there, writing a book?! It's *highly* unlikely that your friend is exercising as intensely as the Belly Fat Free Program recommends. Granted, she may be in the building, but do you really know what she does the whole time she's there?

I know many people who get a little sidetracked when they work out. Maybe they'll do a few exercises then talk with a friend. Or talk to a trainer for a while, read the latest fitness magazine in the locker room, sit in the sauna, or…you get the point. Perhaps they eventually get around to finishing the workout in a couple of hours, but really it would have taken more like 30 to 45 minutes had they remained focused on the task at hand.

This is not to say that all those other things aren't beneficial on some level, but they aren't going to do your body (or mind) as much good as getting a focused, intense workout under your belt, then moving on with the rest of your life. It takes an intense stimulus (workout) to get your muscles to adapt and change shape. But they also need time to recover once the work is done.

Muscles don't get tighter and stronger during the workout; *it's during recovery time when the real adaptations occur.* That's why it's important to do the BFF Resistance Routine every other day, not every day. It's a total body routine, which means that all your major muscle groups are taxed in one workout. So you *need* the day of recovery between sessions.

If your friend really is exercising intensely for long periods of time, then I can guarantee you she is overtraining. And that could also be why she rarely meets her goals. Just because 30 minutes of intense training is good, it doesn't mean an hour or two is better.

Q: *I've reached a plateau. Now what?*

A: Don't fret—with any weight loss program it's pretty common to reach a point where the changes in your body slow down a bit. In the beginning everything you do is new, so you'll probably see some improvements fairly quickly. But then your body adapts to the program, and that's when changes aren't as rapid as we'd like.

So now what? Well, you've got several options:

✔ Add some new movements to the Resistance Routine.

✔ Incorporate new types of Fat-Burning exercise. If you've been walking, try cycling or swimming. Or consider a sport you can do with a friend, like tennis or racquetball.

✔ Try adding one of the scientifically backed supplements from Chapter 8 to accelerate your results from the BFF Eating and Activity Program.

✔ Do the 3-Day Belly Bulge Cleanse that came with your program to get rid of the trapped waste in your digestive system that is weighing you down.

Q: *What if my job requires me to travel? That's always the downfall of my weight loss attempts.*

A: Travel can make staying on some exercise programs difficult, but that's not the case with the Belly Fat Free Program. Everything about the program is portable and flexible.

The BFF Resistance Routine can be done anytime, anywhere. I suggest calling your hotel ahead of time to see if they have an exercise facility. Most places will have *something* you can use, whether it's dumbbells or machines. (If not, just do push-ups, wall squats, abdominal crunches and dips without weight.) And the Fat-Burning Routine is easily adaptable to a hotel pool, treadmill, or stair climber. If all else fails, just get outside and take a walk!

As for the BFF Eating Program, also no problem. Just pack some almonds, fruit, and Belly Fat Free Smoothies and Nutrition Bars so that if you're too busy to sit down to a meal, you'll still have healthy options available to you. If you *can* make it to a restaurant, just ask about low-fat alternatives or find a salad bar with quality protein selections and low-fat dressing. Restaurants like Subway have some decent choices for sandwiches as well. For a free copy of my BFF Fast Food Cheaters Guide, visit: BellyFatFree.com/fastfood.

Q: *I've tried getting into shape countless times. Having a contest goal to shoot for is a little different, but what else should I do to make sure I don't give up this time?*

A: First of all, rest assured you are not alone. Most people who find success through the Belly Fat Free Program have had less-than-terrific results with many other plans. Sometimes the plans themselves are not effective, but often the real problem is a lack of planning. You must decide in advance how to handle the obstacles you will more likely than not encounter as you go. The old adage is definitely true here: If you fail to plan, you're really planning to fail.

In order to avert disappointment, I've assembled the top obstacles that keep many people from experiencing complete success. Then I describe precise coping skills to help you effectively deal with these obstacles. Ready? Okay. Here we go.

Obstacle #1: You don't have time to prepare healthy meals.

> **Coping Skill #1:** Set aside a few hours one night a week (just skip watching TV for an evening) to make large quantities of your favorite healthful meals. Keep some of what you make in the refrigerator, and freeze the rest in plastic containers for later use. You might even consider paying (or persuading) someone to do this for you if you're really crunched for time.

Obstacle #2: You don't have time to eat five mini-meals daily.

> **Coping Skill #2:** If you implement Coping Skill #1 this shouldn't be a problem because you'll have meals to take with you to work. You can also consider using a quality nutrition shake (like the Belly Fat Free Smoothies or the Belly Fat Free Nutrition Bars available at BellyFatFree.com). Having a ready supply of "fast foods" (the good kind!) like nuts, seeds, fruits, low-fat lunchmeat, and low-sugar yogurt is also a great idea.

Obstacle #3: You're tired of eating bland, boring food.

> **Coping Skill #3:** Please remember, you must prepare healthy food you love to eat. That's the only way *anyone* can stick to *any* program for the long term. Otherwise, you'll find yourself constantly bagging your bland and boring meals in exchange for fast food (the bad kind). Check out BellyFatFree.com/Cookbook for *The Belly Fat Free Cookbook,* which offers more than 100 delicious

recipes that will help mix things up and provide some great healthy alternatives for those potentially killer food cravings. More on combating those cravings below.

Obstacle #4: You can't quit eating junk food and you have uncontrollable cravings.

> **Coping Skill #4:** Remove all the junk food and beverages that contain obesity additives from your home (you know where you've got it stashed), and replace these false foods with healthful foods you enjoy eating. When it's out of sight, it's usually out of mind. (Too bad we can't hide all those fast food signs!)

> Another coping skill to practice is making better choices when it comes to food. If you're craving chips, eat pretzels. Make healthy homemade pizza with more veggies and low-fat cheese instead of ordering out. Enjoy baked French fries instead of deep-fried versions. Instead of a chocolate bar, eat some chocolate with 70% to 80% cocoa levels. You can also avoid temptation by making sure the restaurants you visit offer healthy alternatives. You don't want to find yourself debating whether to have the pork rinds or the foot-long hot dog.

> Here's one last tip. To ward off cravings, don't let yourself get hungry in the first place. That's another reason why the BFF Eating Plan includes five mini-meals every three hours. If you never reach the point of extreme hunger you'll find you have more control over your food choices.

Obstacle #5: You're constantly skipping workouts for lack of time.

> **Coping Skill #5:** This obstacle runs deep for many people. The best solution is to plan and prioritize your life. And the truth is, most of us have more time available than we think. For example, not too long ago I met a woman who told me she wanted to get in shape for her

wedding but just didn't have the time. I asked her to keep track of how she spent her time for the next two days in 30-minute intervals.

As it turns out, she was spending almost four hours a day watching TV, surfing the Internet, and chatting on the telephone. Needless to say, with a little time management she found time to exercise in her small home gym.

Here are a few other simple, time-saving ideas. Buy an exercise bench and a variety of dumbbells so you can get a quality workout in at home or in the office. (I have a gym set up in front of my TV that saves me loads of time.)

You can also try working out during your lunch break or getting up and exercising before work. I recommend keeping an extra set of workout clothes in your car in case you forget to pack them one day.

Obstacle #6: Getting off track or getting stuck.

Coping Skill #6: Focus on your written goals to help get you back on track. **Please read this carefully:** While following this program, you *will* need to overcome adversity. You *will* have setbacks. After all, life is not always a bed of roses, and things that we can't anticipate constantly arise.

This is why I had you complete an assignment in Chapter 3 that clearly defined your goal, your compelling reasons to take action, and how to incorporate special visualization techniques to ensure your success. I then asked you to post this assignment somewhere you'd see it and read it out loud twice a day. Remember? (See page 47 for a refresher.)

By doing this, you will continually remind yourself about what you must achieve. So no matter what unexpected event pops up in your life, no matter what setbacks you encounter along the way, with practice and a focused attention to goals, you won't put your dreams on the back burner every time life throws you a curve ball.

Q: *What are some more of the slimming secrets of the men and women featured throughout* Belly Fat Free?

A: These good folks faced the same temptations and challenges we all face, and yet they overcame them and were rewarded by successfully transforming their bodies. And I'll tell you what—they're a lot happier for it.

Because all of these people had tried to lose weight before finding the Belly Fat Free Program, you might wonder what made the difference this time? By answering this question, we can uncover some powerful secrets everyone can use to achieve their own Belly Fat Free transformation.

1. **They didn't let past failures stop them.** Although they had tried many diets before, they didn't give up hope. That's a priceless secret for anyone with an important goal.

2. **They stopped procrastinating.** "I'll start tomorrow" is an excuse that leads…well, nowhere. There's always another tomorrow. "No more excuses!" was the mantra of all these Challenge winners.

3. **They had the courage to face obstacles.** What's so inspiring about these winners is that they all succeeded despite their obstacles. You can, too. The secret is to change your mindset. (See Chapter 3 for details.)

4. **They were 100 percent committed.** None of these successful people achieved their dreams through half-hearted efforts. They didn't take a pair of scissors to the program and cut out parts that were most convenient for them. They embraced all aspects—the healthy eating, the activity, the nutritional supplements, and the positive mindset. If you

want to succeed, embrace the entire Belly Fat Free Program like these winners did.

5. **They joined the BFF Challenge.** Getting involved in the Belly Fat Free Challenge literally propels you to success. The Champions all agreed that the "before" photo required for the contest literally shocked them out of denial and into reality. What's more, entering the contest gave them a powerful goal to strive toward and a deadline to keep them accountable.

6. **They got the support they needed to succeed.** Rarely can someone be successful by him or herself alone. It takes a community. That's why it's no surprise that all of our Belly Fat Free Champions were (and are) extremely active in giving and getting support at BellyFatFree.com.

In case you don't know, BellyFatFree.com is a Web site I created so all of us can help inspire and motivate one another to move toward our BFF goals as a united front. On this Web site you'll find all kinds of interactive tools to help you succeed. You'll also be able to communicate with dozens of other men and women who are involved in the BFF Challenge. (Some members of this Web site have become lifelong friends.) You'll need this type of constant support and inspiration to overcome obstacles and stay accountable for your dreams.

In closing, if you're interested in one-on-one support my "dream team" of Belly Fat Free Coaches, who are experts in guiding men and women to Belly Fat Free success, are taking applications to work with a few select clients. To see if you qualify to work one-on-one with a BFF Coach call 1-877-219-1476 Ext. 601.

BFF Success Story
Jonni: A Mother of Two Rediscovers Her Voice

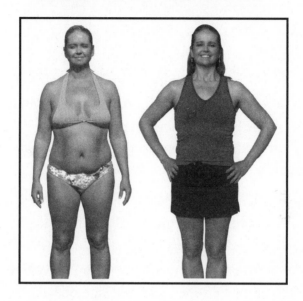

Jonni Isaac was tired of being ashamed of the 30 extra pounds she was carrying around. As she put it, she felt "sluggish, ugly, and old." She certainly didn't feel like the outgoing, confident person her husband had married. Plus, she missed wearing fun, stylish clothes. This mother of two active teenage daughters decided it was time to make a change.

Jonni always had a hard time when it came to her relationship with food. "Chubby" as a girl, she first developed emotional issues with eating in the fourth grade. Jonni says, "Because I was heavy, my mother had to put me in a training bra by the age of eight or nine. The boys did not let me forget that I was so fat I had to wear a bra. When I was 10 or so, I decided I shouldn't climb on top of the fridge to get the peanut butter jar down every day after school. Of course I did it all wrong."

She simply quit eating altogether, enjoying the attention she got from the popular girls who said, "Look at her, she is so skinny!" Jonni soon decided not to eat lunch at all, living mainly on diet soda and apples throughout high school. Her unhealthy behavior continued into college when she would eat a huge breakfast, a salad for lunch, and nothing else for the rest of the day, all the while going to eight or nine aerobics classes per week.

Jonni says that when she resumed eating as an adult, she went right back to the peanut butter jar, spoon in hand. "For me, it was always all or nothing," she explains. It's no surprise, that's how Jonni found herself 30 pounds overweight.

So, armed with the information in *Belly Fat Free*, Jonni began her journey toward transformation. She committed to doing fat-burning aerobic activity every day because, as she puts it, "Women know that those last pounds can be the hardest to lose." She also did resistance training, which helped to boost her metabolism even more and replaced her fat with lean, attractive muscle.

How did the plan work for Jonni? **She lost 17 pounds, but the most impressive statistic is the 28 ½ inches she lost.** She started out wearing a tight size 13, and now she can wear a comfortable size three or four, depending on the style of clothing. That's five pant sizes!

Not only has her shape completely changed, but so has her mental outlook. Jonni says, "I am so much more sure of myself now. I have become a singer in the worship team at church. That wouldn't be so scary if there were 30 or even 20 people singing in front of the congregation with me. But there are only five of us singing, and sometimes only three! Plus, my husband says I walk with more confidence. I don't have to fidget with my clothes when I walk or when I get up and down from sitting. And I know I look good in these jeans. They fit!"

Jonni credits her success to the awesome tools and forums on BellyFatFree.com, which provided her with the motivation and support she needed through her challenge. "The community here is what kept me going. They spurred me on. The coaches are personable and helpful, and several of them I count as true friends."

Belly Fat Free

BFF Charts

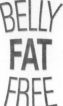

BFF Confidence Booster™

Date:	Goal Weight:	Days To Deadline:

What are you grateful for today?

1. _____
2. _____
3. _____
4. _____
5. _____

What do you admire most about yourself?

1. _____
2. _____
3. _____
4. _____
5. _____

What are your biggest achievements so far in life?

1. _____
2. _____
3. _____
4. _____
5. _____

Before your 12-week deadline, what five things must occur for you to feel successful?

1. _____
2. _____
3. _____
4. _____
5. _____

What five habits will you need to develop to reach your goals?

1. _____
2. _____
3. _____
4. _____
5. _____

Notes: _____

_____

Join our free BFF online community at www.BellyFatFree.com

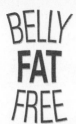

BFF Eating Tracker™

Date:	Goal Weight:	Days To Deadline:

Meal / Time		Source	Met Goal
Mini-Meal One	Protein		☐
	Carb		☐
	Water (oz.)		☐
: AM PM	Supplements		☐
Mini-Meal Two	Protein		☐
	Carb		☐
	Water (oz.)		☐
: AM PM	Supplements		☐
Mini-Meal Three	Protein		☐
	Carb		☐
	Water (oz.)		☐
: AM PM	Supplements		☐
Mini-Meal Four	Protein		☐
	Carb		☐
	Water (oz.)		☐
: AM PM	Supplements		☐
Mini-Meal Five	Protein		☐
	Carb		☐
	Water (oz.)		☐
: AM PM	Supplements		☐

What did I do well today? _____

What will I do even better tomorrow? _____

Join our free BFF online community at www.BellyFatFree.com

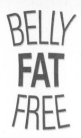

BFF Transformation Tracker™

Date:	Start Time:	Finish Time:

BFF Resistance Routine™	Circuit 1			Circuit 2			Circuit 3		
	Goal Reps	Weight Used	Reps Done	Goal Reps	Weight Used	Reps Done	Goal Reps	Weight Used	Reps Done
Chest Press									
One-Arm Rows									
Seated Overhead Press									
Triceps Kickbacks									
Seated Biceps Curls									
Lunges									
Squats									
Standing Heel Raises									
Double-Leg Stretch									
The Bicycle									

BFF Fat Burning Tracker™	Exercise	Duration	Met Goal
			☐
			☐
Date:			☐

What did I do well today? _____

What will I do even better tomorrow? _____

Notes: _____

_____